The handbook of separation and divorce

T0199796

There is no one in England and Wales whose life is unaffected by marriage breakdown. Yet very few people are well informed about the divorce process or appreciate the wide powers the court has to redistribute property and income after divorce. Those who act on the basis of inadequate information and without the benefit of specialist legal advice can risk impoverishing themselves and their families by accepting less than the court might award them or offering more than the court would order them to give.

The Handbook of Separation and Divorce is principally concerned with the financial consequences of marriage breakdown. It has been written in the shadow of the forthcoming divorce legislation, which is not expected to come into force for two years, but is expected to change the ground for divorce. Emphasising the significance of legal advice, the book refers readers to important decided cases, and, in the appendices, provides a case study of a divorce and a financial relief application.

The Handbook of Separation and Divorce will be invaluable reading for social workers, health professionals and the general public.

Wendy Mantle is a solicitor specialising in family law. She is a member of the Solicitors Family Law Association and has been a member of the Law Society's Family Law Committee. She is a mediator with the Family Mediators Association.

The handbook of separation and divorce

Wendy Mantle

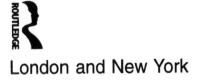

London and New York

First published in 1996
by Routledge
11 New Fetter Lane, London EC4P 4EE

Transferred to Digital Printing 2004

Simultaneously published in the USA and Canada
by Routledge
29 West 35th Street, New York, NY 10001

Typeset in Times by Keystroke, Jacaranda Lodge, Wolverhampton

British Library Cataloguing in Publication Data
A catalogue record for this book is available from the British Library

Library of Congress Cataloging in Publication Data
A catalogue record for this book has been requested

ISBN 0–415–10662–1 (hbk)
      0–415–10663–X (pbk)

Contents

Preface

This book has been written to meet the need of everyone whose marriage may have come to an end. It contains information about the legal processes and financial consequences of divorce and separation.

It does not deal with issues concerning children except insofar as it explains what information the court requires when divorce proceedings are taken; it considers the relevance of the Child Support legislation and the court's powers to deal with cases which are excluded from the jurisdiction of the Child Support Agency. It also contains references to child abduction.

It is hoped that readers will gain sufficient practical information from the book to decide what further steps to take; and those who decide to embark on divorce proceedings should have an idea of the information they need to assemble to assist their solicitors to advise them and prompt the questions they will need to ask them. The crucial importance of obtaining specialist legal advice is underlined for everyone: the repercussions of ill-informed decisions can be disastrous for the lives of the entire families affected.

The book emphasises solicitors' obligation to settle cases where they can be settled and the importance of establishing each person's means consistent with a solicitor's potentially conflicting obligations to clients to obtain a full picture of his or her spouse's finances while ensuring that family assets are not consumed by costs. The book has been written before the form of the government-proposed divorce reform legislation is known, but it refers to expected changes. The new law if passed is not expected to take effect until 1998.

Acknowledgements

It is inevitable that a book which describes areas of law which there is no space to discuss in detail will contain errors of commission and omission. I hope they will not change the balance of any part of the book in a material way. It should be unnecessary to add that any errors that remain are my responsibility.

I owe thanks to the Solicitors Family Law Association for permission to reprint the list of courts in England and Wales which have divorce jurisdiction. I have to thank Gordon Gibb for checking Chapter 3. I am also grateful to the Law Society for permission to reproduce its guidance to solicitors in relation to the pension information and questionnaire reproduced in Appendix 4.

My particular gratitude is due to Gareth Morgan of Dodona for his chapter on benefits and for all the help he and his colleague Clive Trott have given me in writing the chapter on maintenance of children. Their knowledge of the interstices of Department of Social Security and Child Support regulations is unrivalled.

Legal abbreviations

AC	Law reports, Appeal cases
All ER	All England Law Reports
CA	Court of Appeal cases
Ch	Chancery cases
FLR	Family Law Reports
WLR	Weekly Law Reports

Introduction

All happy families are alike but each unhappy family is unhappy in its own way.

This universal truth is recognised by the way the law relating to money and property on divorce works in divorce courts in England and Wales. The courts have discretion to vary property rights and money between divorcing couples as they think fit. Unfortunately, there is no monitoring system to enable solicitors and their clients to establish whether there is a different tariff for the same sort of case in different courts. This has led to calls for hard and fast rules. While it would be helpful to have records there are clear guidelines provided by statute and reported cases. Solicitors who are family specialists are aware of these guidelines when they negotiate agreements to avoid prolonged court disputes.

The purpose of this book is to give anyone contemplating divorce or separation sufficient information to enable them to decide what further advice and information they need and how to get it before coming to a decision. It is accompanied by a warning that contested court proceedings not only consume money which could better be used supporting members of the separated family but they also, by fuelling disputes, use up energy which would be better directed in re-establishing splintered lives.

In 1957 a Church of England Commission on divorce expressed the view that the divorce law should be administered 'with maximum fairness and minimum bitterness'. In the ensuing period social attitudes and changes in the law have improved the climate for separate families but the Church of England's objectives remain an ideal rarely fulfilled. With a marriage breakdown rate of one in three and an unascertainable breakdown rate of cohabitation arrangements the degree of financial and emotional dislocation caused to society is impossible to measure.

This is not, however, a book which blames separating couples for failing to resolve their problems. Nor will it suggest that they should resolve them by ignoring them and continuing to live together. Living together may be an impossible strain for them and, more importantly, their children. In those circumstances it is better for them to part. The parting should be an informed decision reached after advice has been given and considered.

Getting appropriate advice is no easy matter. Legal aid (see Chapter 3) is now available in very few cases as a result of government cuts in eligibility. It was never free; legally aided people who retained a share of their house or other property had always to pay their costs from the proceeds (provided they exceeded £2,500) unless and to the extent that their former partners were ordered to do so. Various sources of help are listed on pp. 233–4.

How to find a solicitor is considered in Chapter 2. It is essential for couples and those advising them, whether in advice centres, the social service departments of local authorities, the courts or parts of the National Health Service, to recognise that the courts require solicitors to attempt to reach a settlement of disputed issues, although this may prove impossible if one or other party takes a different view of what may be the real objective. In a period of just over ten years more than 3,000 solicitors who specialise in family work have joined the Solicitors Family Law Association (SFLA). This organisation was established to encourage negotiated settlement rather than submission to a court order at the end of long and expensive proceedings. Its members subscribe to a code which obliges them to try and reach agreement.

Three different and largely unconnected pieces of legislation have changed the face of family law in the last decade. First the Matrimonial Proceedings Act of 1984 gave courts the power to dismiss a spouse's right to maintenance from a former husband or wife in appropriate cases. It also conferred on courts the power to dismiss a former spouse's right to make a claim against the estate of the other. In consequence wives who would formerly have been able to seek maintenance on a long-term basis subject to variation in that provision when their means or their former husband's circumstances changed, were obliged to establish their inability to support themselves wholly or in part from their own earnings; and many older women who had throughout their marriages been dependent on their husbands were concerned that courts would use their new powers to cut off their maintenance a few years after their divorce.

While it had always been the case that wives who forwent career opportunities while they were married in order to look after their children were meeting social expectations, the new law reflected a change in that attitude in that wives were now expected to find paid work where possible. To some extent the change in the law was the result of a powerful lobby for change from former husbands with second families; to some extent it was the recognition of the increased participation of women in the work force; and to some extent it reflected a change in the attitude of women who had been married who did not wish to be financially dependent if they had opportunities to become self-reliant.

Since 1973 the Matrimonial Causes Act had required the earning capacity of both parties to be considered by the court as one of a number of relevant issues when financial orders were made. Before the 1984 Act it was often a term of a financial settlement that a wife would agree to have her financial rights dismissed. The dismissal was sometimes in exchange for more capital provision if that could be afforded. Earlier, in 1981, the House of Lords gave its approval to the principle of what became known as the 'clean break' where as a result of an agreed settlement or a court order after the 1984 Act came into force neither party would have any continuing financial obligation to the other.

The second major legislative change was the Children Act of 1989. This was partly the product of concern in the public sphere about issues concerning children in the care of local authorities and partly in recognition of the fact, long emphasised by judges and responsible solicitors, that children have rights in relation to both parents, and not the reverse. Orders governing arrangements for the children of divorcing parents were now to be the exception rather than the rule. Approval of arrangements for a child ceased to be a required part of divorce procedure. Arrangements providing for a child to share his or her home with each parent received explicit approval. The Act was non-interventionist and gave children a right to be heard by providing for them to be separately represented.

During the 1980s and 1990s the number of divorces rose from 147,000, to 165,000 a year in 1993. In the meantime the popularity of marriage decreased: there were just under 221,000 first marriages in 1983, falling to just under 182,000 in 1993 (Office of Population Censuses and Surveys), the lowest level since 1889.

While this book was being written the government produced a White Paper entitled *Mediation and the Grounds for Divorce* (1993). The existing law is described in the following chapters but must be read in the shadow of the new proposals. They are the subject of the Family Law Bill which if passed should take effect in 1998 after a pilot study has been carried out. The White Paper anticipates compulsory attendance by would-be petitioners at information sessions followed by mediation from government-approved mediators. Involvement in mediation is likely to be a precondition for receipt of legal aid, except in cases of violence. It also seems likely that couples may be expected to resolve their differences in an agreement for submission to the court without independent legal advice, a prospect which seems calculated to risk future litigation and costs. It may also be intended to discourage couples from separation.

The Family Law Bill will provide for divorce on one ground only – separation involving 3 months for voluntary marriage guidance, and a further 9 months for reflection if there are no children but 15 months if there are children under 18 during which a couple will be expected to resolve all outstanding questions between them with the assistance of the approved mediation organisations. It has been assumed that mediation will take place before lawyers are consulted at all and, perhaps, as indicated above, without their being involved if agreement is reached.

Another aspect of the proposed reform is that there appears to be no clear proposal for abridgement of the 18-month period before divorce so that a rich spouse may be able to rearrange his or her finances advantageously in order to conceal assets which would otherwise form part of a settlement.

One of the consequences of the increase in divorce has been an increase in the number of single parents who became dependent on income support and other state benefits. The Child Support Act 1991 which became law in April 1993 was intended to reduce the cost to the state of separated families by making absent parents (in 90 per cent of cases absent fathers) pay more money for their children. The Act established an administrative system for the assessment of maintenance payable to children. It is run by the Child Support Agency which is a Next Steps Agency of the

Department of Social Security. The Next Steps Agencies of former departments of the civil service are administratively autonomous from their related agencies such as the Benefits Agency but the Secretary of State for Social Security and his ministers are responsible for the administration of the Next Steps Agencies. The Child Support Agency's powers are operated in parallel with those of the courts, which retain jurisdiction for the maintenance of stepchildren, children one of whose parents are habitually resident abroad and children who are over 19 or in full-time advanced education. The court also retains jurisdiction for spousal maintenance, and for capital for spouses and children. The government has recently decided that cases where child maintenance has already been decided by the court will not be taken over by the Agency, as was provided in the original legislation between 1996 and 1997, but will remain with the court for the time being. The new system which is described in Chapter 10 has been the subject of several sets of amending regulations and a new Child Support Act 1995 has made further changes which will take effect when further regulations are introduced in 1996.

The area which now most needs legal change is pensions. Although since 1973 the law has required the court to consider, when making financial orders, benefits which by divorce a spouse would lose the chance of acquiring, the court does not have the power to split pensions; and most pension schemes which provide pensions for a surviving spouse do not provide for a former spouse, however long the marriage may have been. This difficult problem consumes a great deal of solicitors' time and clients' costs in cases where there has been a reasonably long marriage. The Pensions Management Institute published a report entitled *Pensions and Divorce: Report of the Independent Working Group on Pensions and Divorce appointed by the Pensions Management Institute in agreement with The Law Society 1993*. It was hoped that the report would persuade the government to introduce the pension-splitting legislation it recommended. Instead, in the Pensions Act 1995 a new Section 25(b) was introduced into the 1973 Matrimonial Causes Act. This new section imposes on the court a duty to examine the pensions position and gives the court power to impose an attachment order on pension trustees when a pension becomes payable. The regulations under the Act have not yet been published, so it is too early to say how this will affect divorce in cases where pensions are important, but it is likely to add to the complexity of the situation and will probably mean that there will be fewer clean-break cases where there is the possibility of a wife receiving some income by a system described as 'earmarking' from her ex-husband's pension fund.

Perhaps the most exciting, if largely unsung, development of recent years has been the growth of mediation. This developed from the conciliation movement. Its purpose is to enable couples, with the professional help of family solicitors and family counsellors, to resolve their disputes themselves, subject to independent legal advice. The author is a proponent of this method of dispute resolution provided it is used in tandem with independent legal advice and representation where necessary. Of course, litigation will remain the only alternative in cases where one party is intransigent or acts in a way which is not susceptible to joint discussion. But any work concerned with divorce and separation must acknowledge that today's unparalleled complexity of family networks and problems requires an informed and understanding public and a specialised professional legal service.

Chapter 1

Is your divorce really necessary?

Marriage is a contract which imposes on both parties the obligation to support each other financially. In this it differs from cohabitation. But the extent of the obligation is tested only when the marriage breaks down, a divorce is obtained and the parties apply to the court for financial relief.

In order to obtain a divorce, the husband or wife who petitions has to assert that the marriage has irretrievably broken down, and has further to add the evidence that he or she relies upon. The evidence falls into one of five categories. For an immediate divorce evidence on one of two bases can be used. The petitioner can add to the statement that the marriage has irretrievably broken down an allegation of adultery and assert the intolerability of life with the husband or wife. Alternatively, the petitioner can allege unreasonable behaviour, which has to be behaviour which is so intolerable that the petitioner could not be expected to put up with it. In neither case can a petitioner cite the adultery or unreasonable behaviour as evidence of breakdown if he or she has continued living with the respondent for more than six months after learning of the adultery or suffering the unreasonable behaviour.

If neither of these bases is used, couples have to wait until they have been separated for two years from the date of their separation. The fact of separation is evidence of the breakdown provided that the respondent to the petition agrees that a decree shall be pronounced. It is possible, during a period of separation, for a couple to spend time together but that time has to be added to the two-year period and cannot exceed six months.

The same provision applies to the fourth basis for divorce, which is a period of separation for not less than five years. In this case, no consent is required from the other party. In both cases where divorce is based on the evidence of breakdown provided by separation, the respondent can make an application to the court to stop a decree nisi (which is a conditional decree) being made absolute until the financial circumstances of the respondent have been considered by the court. This application is often necessary to protect wives who have always been dependent and who will lose, on divorce, the chance of acquiring a widow's pension in the future (see Chapters 7 and 12).

The fifth, little used, fact as evidence of breakdown is desertion. This means the leaving of one spouse by another for more than two years without reasonable cause. It can mean that the petitioner has either been expelled from the matrimonial home by the conduct of the other or that he or she has been left in the matrimonial home. The bases for divorce are set out in Section 2 of the Matrimonial Causes Act 1973. This Act is the principal piece of legislation providing for divorce (Chapter 6 explains the procedural steps which have to be followed).

The new Family Law Bill will introduce radical changes in the system from 1998, with an 18-month period for reflection between a statement of marital breakdown and an application for a divorce or separation order as the only basis for divorce. In view of the limitations it is expected to introduce (see Introduction) there may be an increase in divorce before the new law takes effect.

The distinction between an unhappy marriage and one which has irretrievably broken down can only be made by those who have already divorced. Ironically, the fact of divorce is not proof that the marriage did irretrievably break down. It is not unknown for unhappily married couples to divorce because their unhappiness is unresolved although the marriage relationship may not have broken down. Conversely, many husbands and wives stay together for financial convenience or because they consider it to be in the best interests of the children even though their emotional relationship has ceased to be of any significance.

Every married individual, or couple if they are able to discuss their problems together, has to consider whether a relationship has ended. In recent years the relevance of their financial condition has usually been at the forefront of their problems. It is essential they should consider whether difficult financial circumstances exacerbate other problems. If there is no prospect of the financial situation being improved they have to consider how divorce will resolve it.

For instance, if a warring couple are in arrears with mortgage payments on their home, a voluntary sale is more likely to produce a better offer than a forced sale by the building society, but it is unlikely that two homes can be purchased with the proceeds. Perhaps debt counselling in this situation should precede marriage counselling.

Matrimonial counselling should enable a couple to decide whether they can bear to live together in an attempt to recreate their relationship. Often there is no question of joint consultation: if one partner has decided to leave, and is convinced that the marriage is at an end, he or she will not necessarily accept the need for counselling. The partner who remains will be in urgent need of counselling in order to learn to accept the situation or to learn how to persist in trying to save the marriage. He or she may however be forced into proceedings to prevent the other from taking unwise financial decisions such as emptying a bank account.

Legal advice should be obtained at an early stage before any final decisions are taken. Divorce is, after all, a legal process. No responsible solicitor or other adviser will recommend that divorce be undertaken lightly because its consequences, unless they can be agreed, may be unforeseeable. Too frequently, couples separate and make separate arrangements without finding out whether the agreed solution is feasible. Of course if a marriage between financially independent partners ends in circumstances where there are no dependent children it may be that that neither wishes to incur the costs of legal advice; and the only significant asset may be a home which is to be sold and its proceeds equally divided. Many eventualities can be anticipated which should be considered and prepared for in advance. It would be unfortunate if, having divorced on an agreed basis, the husband or wife were later to lose work or earning capacity and find that there was no possibility of claiming maintenance from the other. Equally, if a claim for maintenance was made in a petition and was not dismissed later by an agreed order, the later inheritance of money by the other party could result in a financial claim being pursued.

There are limits to what divorce and financial proceedings can achieve. One purpose of early legal advice is to obtain information as to the likely range of settlement which, in each case, it may be possible to expect. If a client is prepared to discuss matters with his or her spouse in an attempt to resolve matters it may be useful to refer the couple to mediation. Mediation is a process designed to help couples resolve their disputes in relation to children and money. There are many different models, some involving one mediator and others two. It can take place before or during the divorce and financial proceedings. It may result in no agreement at all or agreement on some or all issues. Each party should always obtain independent legal advice on the proposed terms of settlement.

Experienced solicitors will provide details of guidelines used by the court in settlement of financial claims, and in cases involving children will be familiar with the different kinds of arrangement which can be made. They should also be able to provide, if given sufficient financial information, details of the likely child maintenance assessment which the Child Support Agency will award in respect of the children. This situation can be very complex where shared arrangements for children are proposed and will often complicate the budget planning of both parties.

It will be reasonable for divorcing couples to expect the same level of information from mediators if the proposed legislation becomes law. But those expectations may be unrealistic unless the new mediators have the same responsibility to their clients as solicitors have, and it follows that they would then be expected to have the same kind of indemnity insurance arrangements which solicitors are compelled to have.

One or both parties to a marriage may be deterred from proceedings because of the uncertain outcome of the financial applications they may make or of their applications in relation to the children; they should always be aware of the time, energy and costs which will be consumed. Separation may be an easier alternative in the short or medium term; divorce after all is not compulsory. On the other hand if, having obtained all the necessary information and advice, it is essential for the well-being of the family and the individuals to proceed, negotiations to lead to a divorce should begin.

Chapter 2

First steps

THE IMPORTANCE OF UNDERSTANDING THE LAW

The prerequisite to action is familiarity with the law and procedure. An outline is set out in Chapters 6 and 7 but information on the substantive legislation referred to at the end of those chapters can be obtained from good reference libraries.

Statutes concerned with matrimonial law, like court decisions on how they apply to different cases, are the centre of a web of legislation on other subjects – housing, insolvency, company law and property law – which, depending on the circumstances, can have a decisive effect on the outcome of matrimonial disputes.

Anyone thinking of permanent separation or divorce has to decide what he or she would like to achieve and establish whether it is possible to achieve those objectives. The fact that legal aid for divorce is now available for many fewer litigants does not mean that legal representation is unnecessary, or that it is safe for one party of a marriage to proceed without representation while the other may be able to pay for advice and representation. But whether someone is eligible for legal aid, or is not eligible and can pay privately (see Chapter 3), or prefers to act for him/herself perhaps with advice from a solicitor from time to time, knowledge of the law is an essential tool.

THE OBLIGATION TO TRY AND SETTLE DISPUTES

Since 1990 solicitors have been obliged to seek a settlement of all issues in dispute between divorcing couples. There are detailed rules providing for the procedure in divorce and related applications, and the Family Division of the High Court provides practice directions which clarify or state how particular matters should be dealt with.

The occasion for issuing the practice direction in Appendix 2 was a case in which the costs consumed by litigation were wholly disproportionate to the assets involved. The direction concludes with these words 'While it is necessary for the legal advisers to have sufficient knowledge of the financial situations of both parties before advising their client on a proposed settlement the necessity to make further enquiries must always be balanced by a consideration of what they are realistically likely to achieve, and the increased costs which are likely to be incurred by making them.'

For many years solicitors specialising in family law had, when appropriate, pursued the goal of settlement if it was necessary to begin financial proceedings in the courts. The Solicitors Family Law Association, founded in 1982, has a code of practice which requires its members to conduct cases in a manner conducive to settlement. This does not mean that in a case where there is violence or where the assets are removed from the country the family specialist does nothing. It is the solicitor's duty to protect the interests of the client in the best way possible. This will often involve a willingness to take assertive action and in an emergency to take action without warning.

Where a case is not settled the courts have very wide powers, which can be exercised when the divorce decree is made absolute. Evidence in the form of sworn documents and disclosure of financial information by each party has to be completed before the court hears the case. In too many instances financial information disclosed by one party, which provides the basis on which court orders are made, is incomplete or inaccurate. The court's powers are exercised on a discretionary basis but within the guidelines discussed in Chapter 7. Its concerns are that each party should have a roof over his/her head and that where possible the children should have continuity of home and school and, if it can be afforded, it may order a clean break which can end the right of either spouse to claim capital or maintenance against the other in the future or against the estate of the other when one of them dies.

A list of the county courts which have jurisdiction to pronounce decrees of divorce and deal with family matters is found in Appendix 3. In London the Principal Registry of the High Court also has jurisdiction to deal with family matters.

The maintenance of most children is dealt with by the Child Support Agency, to which applications for maintenance must be made in all cases where there is no agreement, and no existing court order, and where a child is under 19 or over that age and in full-time but not university education providing he or she has not been married. The Child Support Act does not apply to stepchildren or in cases where one of the parents of the child is habitually resident abroad. In all cases where the Child Support Act does not have jurisdiction the court will continue to deal with child maintenance. However, it is probable that even if written agreement between the parents provides for the maintenance of the child, if a parent wishes to obtain an assessment from the Agency he or she cannot be prevented from doing so.

CHOICE OF SOLICITOR

The satisfactory solicitor is one who will settle a case if appropriate, and adopt and pursue an assertive position where necessary. In the course of proceedings both a conciliatory and an aggressive stance may be necessary at different stages. The choice of representative is more acutely personal than in an action concerning other kinds of dispute. A solicitor who suits one client may be inappropriate for another for reasons which are wholly unconnected with ability and experience. Clients applying for capital and maintenance vary from those at one end of the spectrum who insist on accepting whatever is offered, however short of their needs it may be, to those who will not accept what they are advised is reasonable but prefer to risk not only money but the uncertainty of a contest before a judge to see whether they may get a better result by fighting instead of negotiating.

Clients who have to respond to claims for capital and maintenance vary similarly; there are those who are prepared to impoverish themselves by offering far more than the court would be likely to order, to achieve an immediate settlement; and there are those who will offer far less than the court might award in the hope that their spouses will not bother to contest it.

Solicitors have a duty to try and establish as economically as possible what the overall financial position is: that is, what are the assets, income, debts and liabilities of each of the parties. If a client does not wish a solicitor to press for disclosure of all the relevant financial information it is only right that the solicitor should advise and warn against settling on terms which the client may later regret. Conversely if the client refuses to agree to negotiate as an alternative to litigation the solicitor has a duty to warn the client against the danger of wasted costs. The financial pitfalls of a gamble are set out in detail in Chapter 3. The most costly battles are not necessarily those where there is most financially to lose, but those where one party is determined to fight to the end whatever the net assets may be. The response to this approach may be civilised resistance but this is difficult to sustain in the face of an onslaught of correspondence and applications.

It is also difficult to proceed if the party refuses to recognise proceedings by failing to acknowledge documents, making it necessary for every application to be personally served by an enquiry agent. This procedure greatly increases the costs, which if the case is pursued may be ordered to be paid by the recalcitrant party.

In the maelstrom of doubt and disturbance which most couples suffer when they or one of them decide that their marriage has broken down the decision to divorce is not automatic. Despite the nostrums in the popular press, practitioners are aware that many couples may not divorce when the marriage has in fact ended but may continue to live together for one or more reasons, of which young children and financial security are but two. Sometimes marriages die quietly. It is not unusual for a husband and wife to seek legal advice as to the consequences of divorce and then to draw back and wait for circumstances to change before making a final decision.

It is vital that people whose marriage is in difficulty should be advised that divorce is voluntary, and that there are alternatives. It may be appropriate for a couple to seek counselling first. The first step is usually not to rush to petition for divorce but to consider what options are available. There is no question that anyone is to be relieved from responsibility for the eventual decision, but it is better for everyone to be as well informed as possible about all the likely consequences.

If the decision is to separate or divorce a couple may jointly seek the assistance of a mediator to help them resolve financial and other matters (see Chapter 14). The organisations involved are listed at the end of the book. The model used by one organisation, the Family Mediators Association, usually involves a lawyer mediator and a family mediator who attend a series of one-and-a-half-hour meetings to help the couple work out the terms of settlement. Full financial disclosure is required. The process is entirely confidential as between the parties, their solicitors and the mediators. What transpires cannot be used by one party against the other in court proceedings.

Often couples undertake mediation before taking independent legal advice. Sometimes they take legal advice during the course of the period when they are in mediation. As the leaflet advertising its services says: 'Mediators treat all discussions as strictly confidential except where someone's life or welfare may be in danger. Financial information may be used by either party should there be court proceedings. However, discussions to try to resolve differences are "without prejudice" and therefore legally privileged from disclosure to anyone else.' What this expression means is that neither party can use what has been said in the discussions in open correspondence between solicitors or in court or in affidavits (sworn documents which set out the facts and arguments of the case). Consequently, without prejudice discussions are free from the constraints of open discussions. They enable couples to talk freely about all the possibilities they may need to consider.

The other principal family mediation service provider is National Family Mediation. It has 60 services throughout the country and provides an independent service regardless of ability to pay. The two organisations are being merged and they will be known as the UK College of Family Mediators. The primary focus of National Family Mediation is on children issues, but increasing numbers of its services now offer mediation on all issues arising from separation and divorce according to the same code of practice as the Family Mediators Association.

Mediation is inappropriate if there is a situation of continuing violence or if one party fears, as a result of experience in the relationship, that he or she will be browbeaten.

Whichever course a man or woman takes he or she must ensure that the legal issues which may affect the outcome are identified. It is potentially disastrous if they are not.

There are as many examples as there are failed marriages to illustrate the importance of correct identification of legal issues, and the dangers inherent in the absence of independent legal advice. Those dangers were very clearly set out in a decision of the House of Lords, the highest court of appeal in a case involving Barclays Bank and a Mrs O'Brien (1993 4 All ER). This was a case, like many others, where the husband, a businessman, wanted to remortgage the matrimonial home through the bank. There is always a number of problems inherent in such a situation, since the wife needs to know exactly how her husband's indebtedness will affect the value of the home. The lender needs to ensure that the wife's knowledge is accurate and that she is independently advised. The judgment in this case was that where a wife or cohabitant has signed a mortgage document, has had no independent legal advice, and was misled by her husband into believing that his borrowings were for a much smaller amount than the actual loan secured on the house, the transaction could be set aside. The fact that the bank had sufficient notice of all the circumstances is crucial to the decision. The court held that the obligation of a cohabitant to repay the loan would be enforceable if there had been no misrepresentation and if the lenders had taken reasonable steps to ensure that the cohabitant undertook the new obligation with full knowledge of the facts. It cannot be too strongly emphasised that it is most important for everyone concerned in such a transaction to take advice in order to avoid the problems which arose in that case.

A wife may be asked to agree to increase the mortgage on the matrimonial home and she will want to know how the increased loan will benefit her. Her solicitor may suggest that provided her husband demonstrates that his business needs the cash the bank should agree to the loan being charged against the house on condition that if the marriage breaks down the house will be dealt with as if its value is unaffected. Of course this will not assist if the business fails.

Another very common problem arises where a husband may believe that his wife's friendship with another man is the real reason for her wish that he should leave the matrimonial home rather than her stated reason, which is their present difficult relationship. He will be concerned to know whether he should do as he wants and remain, exacerbating the bad atmosphere between them, or leave for the sake of peace. Either way, he says, the children will suffer. He will want to know whether his claim to a share in the matrimonial home will be affected and whether his continuing obligation to support a dependent wife will mean that, if a long time elapses before there is a divorce, his claim to argue that the house should be sold will be weakened.

A woman may be married to a man who at a difficult time in

their marriage, apparently to reassure her, transferred the valuable matrimonial home into her sole name. It may have no mortgage and the wife may have young children but no job. If, a year later, she finds that her husband's business is in difficulty and he cannot pay his debts she will need to know if the matrimonial home where she and the children live will be sold.

A wife in her forties or fifties who has been financially dependent on a high-earning husband for most of the marriage and is unlikely to become completely financially independent after divorce needs to know whether there is enough capital to give her a home and income and compensate her for the prospective loss of widow's pension from her husband's job and a share of other death benefits. She will want her representative to advise her on whether she will be better off to have continuing maintenance and a potential claim against her husband's estate if he dies before her, or to have a large capital sum with no further maintenance.

THE OBLIGATIONS OF SOLICITORS

The Law Society, the solicitors' governing body, has strictly defined the obligations of solicitors to their clients (Law Society, 1991). These include the obligation to provide terms of business to prospective clients. Many firms have long had this practice and it is essential to ensure that the terms are made clear in writing before or at the first appointment with the solicitor. The most relevant of the terms is the hourly charging rate of the solicitor, legal executive or other fee earner who acts for the client. Rates vary enormously throughout the country and usually depend more on the overheads of the firm than the length of experience of the fee earners. In areas where overheads such as salaries and rent for office accommodation are high the rate will to some extent reflect those overheads. In central London the charging rate for a partner can vary from £100 to £300 per hour. Outside London, £100 per hour is a common charging rate for partners.

Enormous costs which have to come out of the family assets are in no one's interests, although regrettably one party may be forced to incur them if the other refuses to settle. Clients eligible for legal aid will want to know the rate at which their solicitor will be paid, since that payment will be made from what the client recovers in the proceedings. The total charging rate allowed to solicitors will vary from £60 to £70 per hour but some discretion is provided to enable solicitors to be paid at a higher rate in difficult cases. Usually the fact that a case is handled by a solicitor with a great deal of experience makes no difference to the charging rate allowed, so that inexperienced and/or unqualified staff may be more profitable to a firm although of less value to their clients. Where clients cannot get legal aid, they want to establish whether their case is one which they can handle themselves, with assistance where necessary with drafting letters and affidavits and other sworn documents used in financial proceedings. Clients acting for themselves have to file at the court a form called 'Notice of Acting' and send a copy of it to the solicitor on the other side. If later a solicitor is instructed to take over a case entirely he or she files a Notice of Acting with the court and sends a copy to their opposite number. The court has to know who is acting for someone, for it sends notices of hearings and orders made by the court to the solicitor or to the individual acting for him or herself.

The absence of a computer data base of all decisions, whether reached by consent or not, inevitably means that an experienced solicitor competent in negotiations on a without prejudice basis may incur lower costs than an inexperienced one. On a case of moderate complexity it can be useful for an experienced solicitor to be assisted by a less experienced one who can deal with the simpler aspects of the work.

At the outset most solicitors will provide clients with a questionnaire to answer about their financial circumstances and, if they know them, those of their spouse. It will obviously save time if clients prepare their own history of the marriage with a list of relevant financial information and necessary documentation. This can be read by the solicitor, if there is time, before the first appointment, which will shorten the chargeable time spent.

It is essential for clients to feel that their relationship with their solicitor will be a partnership. As far as possible their objectives should be defined at an early stage. There is no point in regarding such objectives as unalterable. The client is paying for advice, which includes advice on alternatives and an appreciation of how changes may force a redefinition of objectives. Thus a man facing retirement whose wife is now living with another man will plan to try and settle her claims in relation to capital only; but if the wife's relationship ends before the settlement is reached or the court decides the issue, the outcome may be different.

Historically, solicitors have distanced themselves from the

public by a sense of their own importance and their need to bolster their confidence in the face of barristers, to whose position as advocates *par excellence* they felt obliged to defer. Some of them increase the sense of distance by the use of portentous language, a characteristic shared by barristers. The recession may have changed the situation by making solicitors more approachable. The majority of family law specialists are keenly aware that claims which can be resolved fairly and quickly create more goodwill than those which cannot. Where they are obliged to pursue claims which will not settle they are conscientious in advising the legally aided client of the amount of costs incurred and in delivering bills regularly to privately paying clients.

Chapter 3

Paying for legal advice and representation

When the emotional and health costs of maintaining a dead marriage become too great for one or both parties to bear, the search for appropriate legal help is inseparable from the search for the means to pay for it.

The first question for someone who is not working, or who is working on a low wage or who is on benefits, is to establish whether the firm he or she consults undertakes legal aid work. For divorce proceedings alone there is no legal aid. There is advice and assistance under what is called the Green Form scheme. Advice involves the steps described below and essentially it requires the petitioner to take documents prepared by the solicitor to the court, documents issued in the name of the petitioner rather than the solicitor. The Green Form scheme, like the legal aid scheme, is administered by the Legal Aid Board, a body independent of solicitors. Eligibility for Green Form advice and assistance depends, like legal aid itself, on a capital and income test. The capital limit is £1,000 if the client has no dependants, rising to £1,535 if he or she has two dependants. It is available to people whose disposable income – allowing for deduction of income tax, national insurance and income support allowances for children and dependent relatives – is less than £70 per week. No contribution is payable for Green Form advice.

The form for advice and assistance is completed at the first interview. Its scope enables the solicitor to do £137.25 worth of work, which at Green Form rates means three hours at £45.75 per hour. The solicitor should be able to take instructions about the history of the marriage, draft a divorce petition, help complete a legal aid application for any proceedings in relation to money or children or in relation to any injunction proceedings which it may be necessary to take. The petition and the statement of arrangements for the children, along with extra copies, will be given to the client to file with the marriage certificate at the local divorce county court. Later, when the petition has been acknowledged by the completion of an acknowledgement of service form by the other spouse, the court sends a copy of it to the assisted person and the solicitor prepares an affidavit for the petitioner to swear. This confirms the truth of the contents of the petition, subject to any corrections, and provides certain additional information (described in Chapter 6). The affidavit is sworn before another solicitor and, with a form called 'request for directions', lodged at the court.

It is not necessary for someone receiving Green Form advice to pay the court fee of £80 on the filing of the petition nor the fee of £20 which is payable when a written application is made to make a decree nisi of divorce a decree absolute. If complications arise under the Green Form scheme a solicitor may be able to obtain an extension to give further advice. An applicant for assistance whose income is over the limit will have to pay privately.

The rates of solicitors vary according to location, the experience of the solicitor and his or her reputation. The most experienced are not necessarily the best, and the cheapest may not be inexperienced, but when charging, more experienced solicitors will cost more than newly qualified solicitors, and solicitors cost more than trainees. However, more experienced solicitors may do the work more quickly and may adopt an overall approach that will lead to less tension and lower costs. What no solicitor can do is to control the conduct of the case unilaterally. If opposed by a solicitor who is determinedly litigious or if his or her client will not try to compromise in order to achieve a settlement, costs will inevitably increase. If junior staff are employed they should be strictly supervised. The partners of a firm are professionally liable for negligence, that is, failing in their duty to their clients, with the result of loss or damage. This liability extends to liability for the work of their staff. The Solicitors Professional Indemnity Fund is responsible for meeting damage or loss and the cost of indemnity insurance is one of the highest overheads of every firm.

A client may be ineligible for Green Form advice but eligible for legal aid. The lower capital limit for legal aid is £3,000 and the upper capital limit is £6,750. The lower income for disposable annual income is £2,294 and the upper £6,800 per annum. At the lower limit no contribution for legal aid will be payable. Disposable income here means the income remaining after allowances for dependants are taken into account, the level of those allowances being the same as for income support (see Chapter 10). Thus a woman whose net income after tax and national insurance is £8,000 per annum and who has two children aged 9 and 12 will have a disposable income of £5891.40 per annum, so will be eligible. If a client may be eligible for legal aid he or she should be so advised and an application submitted. In appropriate cases an emergency application can be lodged, sometimes in advance of completion of the complex form for ordinary legal aid.

The most important factor to bear in mind is that legal aid has always been a loan, and since 1988 has been an interest-bearing loan. It has to be repaid from assets which are said to be 'recovered or preserved' in the proceedings. The only cases in which the loan question is irrelevant are those where a husband and wife have no assets in dispute, where for example their home is rented and they have no significant possessions. A solicitor is obliged to explain that costs are usually met by the Legal Aid Board but will be paid by the client not only from the contribution to costs which will be made on a monthly basis to the Legal Aid Board throughout the proceedings but from the client's share of money or property received from the other party's assets. The first £2,500 of money or property is exempted from the charge for costs. It may also be the case that the other party, if not legally aided, may be ordered to pay the costs or a proportion of them.

In London a solicitor is paid £39.00 per hour for legally aided work, but a higher rate can be sought in cases of exceptional difficulty, and a higher rate in Children Act cases. At this level the cost burden for a client is lower than if he or she paid privately, perhaps by borrowing.

Whether or not a client is legally aided the costs are taxed, that is to say assessed by the court at the end of the proceedings. In the past it has been of great concern to solicitors doing legally aided work that even if an order for costs has been obtained against an opponent, an opponent would have to pay those costs only at a legally aided rate. Since 1994 this has ceased to be the case so there is no purpose to be served by a privately paying opponent of a legally aided litigant conducting the case in a way which increases the costs: he or she may have to pay for them at a much higher rate at the end.

The costs of divorce proceedings are usually awarded against a respondent if the petition is based on evidence of unreasonable behaviour or adultery, but these costs are unlikely to be high compared with disputes about children or property. If the costs are not agreed they will be taxed by the court.

The costs of a financial application will be principally the costs of work involved in correspondence, negotiations, the obtaining of financial information, the preparation of affidavits and the collation of documents for the hearing so that all the relevant information is before the court. Costs can be enormously increased by the need to apply to the court for orders in the course of the case to force disclosure of items of relevant information or to ensure that a case is fixed to be heard when one party is dragging his or her feet.

The Notice of Application on forms M11 or M13 for financial relief which begins at this stage attracts a court fee of £30. Affidavits are filed without incurring court fees. The expenses or disbursements likely to be incurred by the solicitors may be for work by investigative accountants, in relation to valuations of companies, or perhaps for accounts and valuations of properties by surveyors. If expert advice is necessary in legally aided matters it is essential to obtain authority from the Legal Aid Board beforehand, otherwise the solicitor may find that he or she has to meet that cost personally from what is recovered by way of costs.

A matter may be resolved before it is heard. If so, costs will be one of the terms to be agreed. Frequently, after a case has been contested and the parties reach an agreement to avoid a hearing there is an agreement that there should be no order as to costs. A judge at the end of a contested hearing may also make no order as to costs. There are many varieties of order. Where it is necessary to make an application for a financial questionnaire to be answered, the spouse making the application will seek costs against the other. It may be necessary to take steps to obtain or enforce orders in relation to affidavit or other evidence. Where the applicant has merit on his or her side, costs may be awarded in his or her favour or they may be 'reserved'. In that case an order for them must be asked at the eventual hearing.

Thousands of pounds can be spent on a case and solicitors should advise their clients periodically of the amount of costs being incurred, whether they are legally aided or paying privately. The amount of assets in dispute should always be borne in mind. Although disproportionate costs should not be incurred, this advice is difficult to follow when an opponent obstructs the conduct of a case by behaving unconstructively.

In the case of privately paying clients a sum of money will usually be asked for on account of costs at each stage of the work and bills will be delivered regularly throughout the case. The solicitor must provide terms of business initially which will set out the arrangements for the payment of costs. The client may choose to represent him or herself with help from a solicitor, as described in Chapter 2. As the date for trial approaches the client may decide that he or she would prefer to be represented by a detached professional. But the most useful course to adopt, whether represented or not, is to obtain advice when all the relevant financial information is available in order to form a view as to the kind of offer to make. In cases where the financial facts are known this decision can be made early on provided adequate consideration is given to the factors which the court takes into account (see Chapter 7). The offer should be made in a letter headed 'without prejudice save as to costs' so that it cannot be referred to in open correspondence. Such an offer is described as a Calderbank offer, after the name of a case in which the device was first used.

There are of course cases where there is nothing to be lost by making plain in the affidavit evidence filed at the court what an applicant or respondent's position is; and the terms offered or the terms which he or she is prepared to accept can then be set out in the affidavit.

The value of a sensible offer, open or without prejudice, is that it can protect the party making it from payment of the subsequent costs of the other party. If the offer is rejected and if the order made by the court is not as favourable to the other party as the offer would have been, the party who made the offer can seek costs from the date the offer was made. Thus if a husband offers a wife three-quarters of assets worth £500,000, consisting of a house and some investments, for a clean break in relation to capital and maintenance and the court awards the wife two-thirds, the judge will be asked by the husband's solicitor for an order that his costs from the date he made the offer be paid by his wife. Costs are a matter entirely in the court's discretion and because the outcome is uncertain each litigant has to budget for meeting his or her costs as the case progresses. Where at the end of the case, having paid his or her own costs throughout, a litigant is ordered to pay the opponent's costs he or she may well have to sell some of the assets recovered in order to do so.

The risks for legally aided clients and privately paying ones are the same. The legal aid bill, if paid by a legally aided litigant, must be met from any assets recovered or preserved in the proceedings. Thus if the litigant receives half the value of the former matrimonial home which was his or her's anyway the same rule will nevertheless apply because the property is held to have been 'preserved'.

If in the above example the court is not prepared to order a clean break because the wife has no established earning capacity or because three-quarters of the assets would not give her sufficient capital to meet her future needs, it may be that continuing maintenance will be ordered but less capital will be transferred and an order for costs or part of the costs may be made against the husband. As Chapter 7 makes plain, the court's concern in ensuring that the parties are ready for a hearing is also intended to concentrate their minds on costs. The judge requires to know the details of all the costs which have been incurred to the date of the hearing – that is, those which come under the heading of standard costs which are attributable to the correspondence and work done in connection with the other side – and those costs which are incurred in relation to the solicitor dealing with his or her own client. It is very rare that an order for all the costs, that is to say indemnity costs, is made. More usual is an order for payment of costs on the standard basis or an order that a contribution of a fixed sum be made to the other's costs.

Of course where a party is legally aided an order for costs is unlikely if the opponent is also legally aided. However, there is an exceptional provision (Section 17 Legal Aid Act 1988) under which a legally aided person may be made liable for the costs of his or her opponent provided the sum of costs he or she is ordered to pay is 'a reasonable one for him to pay having regard to all the circumstances, including the financial resources of all the parties and their conduct in connection with the dispute'. This means that liability for costs is imposed on a legally aided litigant only when it seems appropriate to the court because he or she is not without financial resources and his or her conduct is in the court's view indefensible. More commonly an order for costs can be made against a legally aided party on the basis that it is not to be enforced without leave of the court.

For clients who own no property the legal aid charge is not a threat. The difficulty for the clients may be the selection of an experienced solicitor within easy travelling distance, a factor likely to be an increasing problem for clients outside large towns since it is only in large towns that solicitors franchised by the Legal Aid Board will be practising. For those above the legal aid limit the problem is to finance costs from highly stretched income, or borrowing on terms which are realistic, given that the final costs cannot be known. It is possible to insure against divorce costs provided the policy is taken out before any question of divorce arises, but the premiums are likely to be high, given the high risk of divorce.

The costs process is unimaginably tedious for clients and practitioners. Detailed costs rules provide for the preparation of bills in an archaic form by a specialist cost draftsman. Legally aided clients are entitled to see copies of their solicitors' bills and be present when they are 'taxed' by the court, as the assessment procedure is called. This procedure is undertaken by a court employee called a taxing officer, who will not conduct a taxation hearing unless a bill is opposed. Where there is an order for one party to pay the other's costs a hearing must take place in which the cost of each item of work will be considered and may be challenged. When the taxation process is completed, with or without a hearing, an order for costs is prepared and sealed by the court. This is called a taxing certificate in the case of bills to be paid by the Legal Aid Board. It shows a breakdown of the costs: what the solicitor is to be paid, the amount of the disbursements incurred, the amount of barristers' fees and VAT. There will be a separate order against any party ordered to pay those costs or part of them. That order will state how much is to be paid, and in the case of legally aided bills enforcement is undertaken by the Legal Aid Board Recovery Department.

For enforcement of these costs reference should be made to Chapter 17.

Chapter 4

Separation

Divorce simply dissolves the legal contract between the parties and it is usual to resolve financial issues between a couple at the same time, invoking the powers of the court to vary property rights if they cannot be resolved by agreement. This means that the ownership by a husband or wife of a house, shares or money in a building society or bank can be varied by the court when it decides how the financial claims are to be met.

SEPARATION WITHOUT AGREEMENT

Separation is often an established fact before either party takes legal advice as to its consequences for the marriage. Absence of information about the consequences may put the party who has left at a disadvantage. It might have dire consequences where one party has resources which are spirited abroad and have disappeared by the time divorce proceedings are taken.

The cost of separate living is greater than the cost of living together but any attempt to return to the matrimonial home may cause further problems, such as an application to oust the returning partner. The time which has elapsed since the separation began is a factor which the spouse who remains in possession of the house may wish to use to bolster his or her position, particularly if children are involved.

SEPARATION BY AGREEMENT

It is often the case that couples separate by agreement so that they will be able to divorce when two years have elapsed from the date of their separation. If financial matters are not resolved in an agreement made at the time of separation or shortly afterwards they will be resolved after the divorce (see Chapter 7). The court exercising its powers to vary property rights takes into account the financial circumstances of the parties at the time of its decision. One of the parties may have changed jobs or inherited a substantial legacy, or rearranged his or her financial affairs in such a way as to present a very different financial picture from the one which would have applied if the divorce had taken place earlier.

There are several benefits for couples who negotiate a separation agreement. First, they may wish to make financial arrangements based on an immediate division of their capital or provision for the proportion of home and money which each will have. They may also wish to ensure that arrangements for paying for children are recorded and that there is no dispute about where the children are to live and how much time they will spend with each partner. It is usual when providing for future housing arrangements and spousal and child maintenance to record the couple's intentions, and the terms of the agreement become the terms of an agreed order when the divorce takes place. The reason why legal advice is desirable is to ensure that each party has given full financial disclosure to the other so that the agreement is made in full knowledge of the overall position. Otherwise the agreement could be set aside.

There is no guarantee that, after an agreement has been made, the parties will not fight over financial matters or the children in the divorce proceedings, but it is less likely; if a financial application is made because one party's circumstances have wholly changed, the other would ask the court to take account of the separation agreement as a factor in determining the issues. The effect of a separation agreement is that while the parties remain married they are relieved of the obligation to live together.

The alternative to separation is immediate divorce. This requires allegations of unreasonable behaviour or adultery (see Chapter 1). Both are likely to engender or perpetuate bad feeling at a time when emotions are at their most volatile. Disputes over children and money are likely to be exacerbated and the costs increased. In 1991 in England and Wales there were 158,745 divorces, of which only 18.6 per cent were based on the evidence of separation of two or five years, 46.4 per cent on the basis of unreasonable behaviour and 28.3 per cent on the evidence of adultery.

The government's Green Paper, *Mediation and the Grounds for Divorce* (HMSO 1993) and its subsequent White Paper *Looking to the Future* (Commd 2799) have already been mentioned. In the first the government invited comments on proposals for reform of the law based partly on the Law Commission's recommendations that there should be one basis for divorce: the ground would be the irretrievable breakdown of the marriage. The evidence would be the view that one or both consider the marriage to be at an end and remain of that view during a 12-month period for reflection and that the issues between them should be worked out during that period.

One of the problems about separation, and the reason why it is relatively little used, is that poorer couples, particularly women with children, cannot afford it. The proposal that people should be able to divorce even if not separated and without having to blame the other is expected to be the cornerstone of reform of the divorce process. Obviously there will continue to be cases where parties want to separate and make their arrangements first where they can afford to live separately.

A DECREE OF JUDICIAL SEPARATION

An alternative to divorce is judicial separation proceedings where one party may not wish the marriage tie to be dissolved, perhaps for religious reasons or for the practical reason that a possible future entitlement to widow's pension would be lost on divorce and no proposals have been made or perhaps cannot be made to compensate the wife for the loss. A decree of judicial separation is sought on the same evidence as divorce, the wording of the petition differing only in the 'relief' which is sought; the person seeking the decree, the petitioner, does not 'pray' – as the current terminology archaically requires – for a divorce, but for a decree of judicial separation. The remedies available to divorcing couples are available to couples with judicial separation decrees, with two important differences. First, even though capital provision can be made by the court the order will not necessarily be a final one, as a financial order at the end of the divorce process would be. Secondly, it is not possible for the court to dismiss either party's rights to claim provision from the other's estate after his or her death; this is a common provision in financial proceedings following divorce, usually where a wife does not receive maintenance after the divorce (Inheritance (Provision for Family and Dependants) Act 1975).

A decree of judicial separation may be replaced by a decree of divorce when five years have elapsed from the date of the separation. The consent of the unwilling party does not have to be obtained.

Chapter 5

Emergency remedies

Some emergency remedies can be obtained without divorce proceedings. These include orders for personal protection of a spouse and children and orders in relation to property.

As a result of the abandonment by the government of the Family Homes and Domestic Violence Bill 1995 in November 1995 the law in respect of personal protection and occupation of the family home is still governed by the Domestic Violence and Matrimonial Proceedings Act 1976 in relation to married couples and unmarried couples who cohabit or have cohabited in the six months prior to an application to the court. In relation to other family members personal protection is obtained by applying for the common remedies of assault and trespass in the county courts. The Family Homes and Domestic Violence Bill was drafted by the Law Commission and its proposals had been considered by a Home Office select committee in 1993. It had the support of all parties and was introduced in the 1994–95 session of Parliament in the House of Lords under the public law procedure. It would have simplified and streamlined the present position by providing a single set of remedies to a wider category of what are called 'associated persons' – parents and children as well as spouses and cohabitants – and would have lengthened the periods during which victims of violence could occupy the homes in which they had lived. It would also have provided for the removal of an abuser of a child from the home, a more appropriate remedy than that which now obtains, namely the removal of the child by the local authority from the home occupied by the abuser. The principal provisions of the abandoned bill have been reinstated in the new Family Law Bill. What follows is a description of the current hotchpotch.

PERSONAL PROTECTION

Both magistrates' courts and those county courts which are divorce courts have power to make orders to prevent a party to a marriage from harassing the other or behaving violently. The Domestic Proceedings in Magistrates' Courts Act 1978 first enabled magistrates' courts to make orders similar to injunctions made in the county courts. The Act applies only to married people and does not include harassment unless violent threats are made. An application, which can include not only the children of the parties but children who have been treated as children of the family, can be made at the same time as an application for maintenance.

An applicant makes a complaint orally or in writing to the magistrates' court so that a summons can be issued. It is possible for a court to make a protection order without serving the summons on the spouse who is the respondent if there is danger of injury to the applicant or the children. Such an order is called an expedited protection order. The order is only effective when served on the other party and lasts for 28 days or until the case is heard.

An exclusion order excluding the violent partner from the family home for a defined period of time can be made in the magistrates' court in certain circumstances. It does not affect the property of either party and, as in the High Courts, is not a long-term remedy, lasting for a maximum period of six months.

If the respondent, usually the husband, against whom the order is made breaks the terms of the order and returns to the home the order can be enforced. If the order has a power of arrest attached to it a copy of it will be given to the local police station and the respondent will be arrested by the police and brought before the court within 24 hours of his arrest. He may be ordered to be remanded in custody for up to three days in a police station or eight days in prison.

If there is no power of arrest attached to the order the applicant applies on oath to a justice of the peace for a warrant. A justice of the peace has to have reasonable grounds for believing there has been a breach of the order if a warrant is to be issued.

If there is harassment and no threat of violence it is possible for the person suffering it to apply to the county court under the Matrimonial Causes Act 1973 if divorce proceedings have been or are about to be instituted, but if there is violence and the parties are living together as man and wife, whether or not they are married, the application can be made under the Domestic Violence and Matrimonial Proceedings Act 1976. The application is accompanied by an affidavit, a sworn statement setting out the history of the behaviour complained of. The order obtained is called a 'non-molestation order'.

If there is serious violence or threat of violence an application can be made to the court for an order without serving the application on the other party, the respondent. This is an ex-parte application. In these circumstances application can also be made for a power of arrest to be attached to the order. When made, the order has to be served on the respondent and if a power of arrest is attached to it a copy of it has to be lodged at the appropriate police station as with the same kind of order in the Magistrates' Court. With the order is served a summons to appear in court to answer the allegations at a later date, usually between a week and ten days later. On that date the respondent may offer the court an undertaking, that is a solemn promise, not to molest the applicant or be violent even if the allegations are denied. The respondent is bound by this undertaking and the new order will not have to be served upon him. But if he breaks its terms the order has to be served so that an application can be made to commit the respondent to prison for breaking the order. The application has to be supported by an affidavit setting out what has happened.

If the violence she has suffered is such as to make it impossible for a woman fearful of her husband to return to the matrimonial home she can apply after obtaining a non-molestation order from the court without service of the application on the husband for an ouster order to exclude him from the home. If made on the return date appointed for the husband to appear in court this order would exclude the husband for a limited period or until further order, usually three months later, from the matrimonial home (Matrimonial Homes Act 1983 Section 1(iv)). The purpose of the three-month period is to enable the partner to seek other remedies to resolve the situation. For example in divorce proceedings the applicant may seek a transfer of property order under Sections 23 and 24 of the Matrimonial Causes Act. If the parties do not wish to obtain an immediate divorce they may take other steps to determine their entitlement to a share in the matrimonial home. They might seek an order for sale under the Married Women's Property Act 1882 or, if no immediate sale is feasible, a declaration of their interests in the property under the Law of Property Act 1925 (Section 30). These questions are considered further in Chapter 9.

The remedies provided by the new Family Law Bill can be obtained not only by people who are or have been married to each other but also by cohabitants or former cohabitants or by those who live or have lived in the same household, or are relatives, are parents of a child or have parental responsibility for a child.

The new Bill will provide that a spouse who does not have a beneficial, that is an enforceable, right to occupy a home does have a right to occupy it while the marriage subsists, as was provided by the Matrimonial Homes Act 1983, and if the house is subject to an assured tenancy, that is to say a tenancy in the private sector whose terms are defined, the spouse must occupy it 'as his only or principal home'. The right to occupy is now called 'matrimonial home rights'.

The Family Law Bill, like the abandoned Family Homes and Domestic Violence Bill, will give the court power to make occupation orders which could regulate the occupation by either party or require one of them to leave the home. The duration of the orders would have been up to six months if the applicant does not have an entitlement to occupy the property, but could be extended. If the applicant is a cohabitant and not a spouse only one six-month extension will be granted. It will be possible for the order to include provision for repair and maintenance of the property and provide for payments to the other spouse for accommodation.

The new Bill provides, as the present law does, for non-molestation orders. Undertakings can be accepted by the court from the respondent not to repeat the behaviour unless there is already a power of arrest attached to an order. The terms in relation to bringing a respondent before the court would be the same as before.

An application may be initiated in a magistrates' court by an individual or her solicitor, since these are treated as family proceedings, but magistrates' courts may decline jurisdiction if it is more convenient for an application to be dealt with in a different court.

Although the key feature of the anticipated divorce reform legislation is a period of one year for reflection following a statement of breakdown it will be required that couples resolve outstanding issues between them before a petition can be filed for divorce. It is not clear whether emergency reliefs of the kind described can be obtained within the period, although the law relating to emergency relief on financial matters remains the same. However, it appears that the kinds of order discussed below, to protect property, may not be available. In that case, as suggested in Chapter 1, it may be possible in the future for people of means to rearrange their finances in such a way as to avoid the rigours of the present law, by concealing how they have disposed of their capital.

ORDERS TO PREVENT PROPERTY, WHETHER MONEY OR ASSETS, BEING TRANSFERRED OR SOLD OR MOVED ABROAD

At present orders can be made under Section 37(2) of the Matrimonial Causes Act 1973. This Act is the principal one dealing with the law on marriage breakdown and if the court is satisfied that one party intends to defeat an ancillary relief claim by dealing unilaterally with property under his or her control it can make an order restraining the disposal of the assets, setting aside transfers already made.

For such an order to be made the applicant must show that there already exists an application for ancillary relief, which may be in the petition or the answer to it. The court (see Chapter 6) must be satisfied that the disposal of the asset has taken place or is about to be made and that this is intended to defeat the claim of the petitioner.

An order cannot be obtained if the disposition is in a will or codicil (see Chapter 16) nor if it is to a third party who has no knowledge of the application. Thus if one party sells valuables to a jeweller who has no knowledge of the situation, the jeweller paying the correct price should not suffer by being compelled to restore the goods. It would be otherwise if the jeweller were in collusion with the party selling the goods. Similarly a bank through which funds were transferred abroad would be protected unless it acted in bad faith and had had notice of the application.

The order is made ex-parte, that is without notice to the respondent, in the first instance to ensure that the respondent is not able to remove the assets from the jurisdiction. On making the order the court then appoints a time for an inter-partes hearing, for which notice is served on the respondent so that he or she can apply to set aside the order. The application is made to a district judge and supported by an affidavit describing the property and the need for an order. On the date of the hearing of which the other party has notice the court will consider his or her affidavit evidence. This may point out that the property removed was placed abroad in the normal course of business and that sufficient property remains in England and Wales to satisfy any order the court subsequently makes.

The difference between Section 37 orders and those which are described as Mareva injunctions is that the latter can be made where the parties are not married and can be made after the final order has been made. They can also be made to prevent assets which are the subject of an order being disposed of before an order has been executed. Any third party involved who is aware of the existence of such an order is in contempt of court and applicants must therefore make sure that the orders are served on relevant banks and third parties. Common to applications for both kinds of order is the requirement that the applicant undertake to be responsible for any damage which is caused to the respondent as a result of the making of the order. This requirement underlines the gravity of the procedure.

Chapter 6

The divorce process

The present law on divorce is largely contained in the Matrimonial Causes Act 1973. This provides the ground for divorce and the financial orders which can be made when a divorce takes place, and sets out the factors to which the court has regard in making these orders.

Divorce proceedings can begin when a couple have been married for at least one year.

Divorce petitions are relatively simple documents and can be bought at law stationers'. Where couples have had short marriages, have no children and have agreed on how their assets should be divided there is no reason why they should not undertake the process themselves, provided they each obtain advice as to their respective financial situations and the desirability of concluding matters with an agreed order which will have the effect of dismissing their financial claims against each other for the future.

Reference has already been made to the fact that although the one ground for divorce is the irretrievable breakdown of the marriage, it can be evidenced by one of five facts (Chapter 2). Because the majority of divorcing couples cannot afford to wait for a divorce based on two years' separation, it is more usual to allege unreasonable behaviour or adultery. Happily, in the latter case, it is no longer necessary to name the third party. If it is important to proceed on the evidence of unreasonable behaviour and agreement has been reached on financial questions, it is tactful to ensure that the spouse who is the subject of the allegation sees the document in advance. Allegations which are unexpected can stoke up fires of bitterness.

The behaviour complained of should not consist of a mixture of trivial and serious allegations. The list should be confined to a few incidents, or aspects of behaviour, which will indicate to the district judge of the county court where the petition is filed that the behaviour was such that the petitioner who complained of it should not have to live with the other party.

The other evidence of breakdown consists of two years' separation or five years' separation or desertion. The first is granted provided the respondent gives his or her consent by personally signing the acknowledgement of service form which the court sends with a copy of the petition to the respondent. The second does not require consent; in both cases the petitioner must provide as precisely as possible the date of separation.

The third is desertion. This evidence of irretrievable breakdown is little used. Its significance is that it is an allegation that one party has left another without reasonable cause for a period of two years. The defence to such an allegation if it were pursued may be that the respondent expressed the wish to return but the offer was rejected. The effect of such an offer could put the petitioner in desertion.

CONTENTS OF PETITION

The printed forms of petition leave blank spaces for insertion of details of where the marriage took place, the address where the parties last lived together, their present addresses, their occupations, and a statement as to whether each of them is resident or domiciled in Great Britain. The details of where the marriage took place have to be stated in the same form as in the marriage certificate, which has to be filed at the court with the petition.

The court only has jurisdiction to dissolve marriages where one of the parties has ordinarily been resident in England or Wales for one year or lives here permanently, or where one party describes themselves as having their permanent home here; this is the meaning of 'domicile'. Wherever in the world a petitioner lives, if he or she has a spouse living ordinarily in Britain, for example on a three-year contract, he or she can petition here.

The petitioner has to provide details of the place of birth of the children of the family who are under 18, or their number and the fact that they are over that age. The children include stepchildren or those who may be regarded as children of the family. It is also necessary to state whether any other children have been born since the marriage. It is necessary to state in all cases (whether or not there are children of the marriage) if an application has been, or will be, made to the Child Support Agency.

A statement has to be made as to whether any other proceedings have been taken by either of the parties in any other court or the same court. Any old petitions filed in England and Wales or elsewhere in the world not proceeded with, or proceedings in the magistrates' court, would be relevant, as would any current proceedings brought under any other laws, for example the Married Women's Property Act 1882.

In a petition where divorce is sought on the evidence of adultery a statement to this effect is followed by particulars of the association and the dates and places where the petitioner knows or believes that adultery has occurred. It should be ascertained in advance whether adultery will be admitted by the respondent. It is not sufficient that the petitioner believes or suspects that adultery has occurred: he or she must know it is so. A further requirement is that the petitioner can use this ground only if the couple live together in the same household after the knowledge was acquired for a period of less than six months. If the six-month period has expired or if the petitioner merely suspects from the respondent's behaviour that adultery has occurred, the conduct giving rise to the behaviour may be cited as a example of unreasonable behaviour.

Where evidence of unreasonable behaviour is required the complaints should be reasonably precise, with dates if possible where particular incidents are the subject of complaint. In cases of unreasonable behaviour also, the petition may not be filed if the couple have lived together for more than six months after the last incident complained of.

Petitions end with a request (or prayer, as it is still archaically called) for divorce, for costs to be paid by the respondent and for financial relief. Costs are not sought when the evidence on which a divorce is sought is the parties' separation for two or five years. Part of the negotiations may have resulted in an agreement that no order for costs will be sought, or the other party may have agreed to pay them. The costs of an undefended divorce are a few hundred pounds and although this is a significant sum to most people it is very much less than the thousands of pounds that can be spent on separate financial proceedings.

Several financial claims are set out in a petition. First, there is a claim for a wife petitioner for maintenance or 'periodical payments', as continuing maintenance payments are called. This is followed by a claim for secured provision: this means that the court may be asked to provide that maintenance is secured on an asset such as a property so that if the money is unpaid the property can be sold to pay the arrears. There will also be claims for capital. These are in two forms. One is for lump sums and the other is for property adjustment. A lump sum simply means a capital amount. Property adjustment means an order in relation to the property either or both parties own which may be transferred to one or other of them on certain terms. Capital claims can be made for children of the family whether or not they are within the jurisdiction of the Child Support Agency. The Agency deals only with maintenance on a weekly basis. The usual order sought by husbands is for lump sum and property adjustment. Maintenance is a less likely claim, but it can be made and is sometimes ordered in husbands' favour.

The purpose of leaving in a petition general financial claims is to ensure that all or some of them can be pursued if necessary. Even if it is later agreed that all financial claims shall be dismissed they have first to be made so that they can be dismissed. A request for financial relief in a petition is considered to be a claim.

Where there is agreement about dismissal of claims the respondent has also to make a claim if he or she has not already done so, and this is called 'an application for dismissal purposes only' (see Chapter 7).

The petition has to be signed by a solicitor or the petitioner if he or she is not represented by a solicitor. The address at which the respondent is to be served with a petition must be placed at the end. If the respondent does not have a solicitor it will be the home address, wherever that may be. A party living outside England and Wales is obliged to find an address in the jurisdiction where notices of applications and proceedings can be served. An address for service is one to which court documents and solicitors' correspondence may be sent in the expectation that it will be received.

Where a couple have children a statement of proposed arrangements for them has to be filed with the petition. The Children Act 1989 which became law in 1990 changed the vocabulary used in relation to the claims that parents make in respect of children. The philosophy underlying the Act was that a child has a right to two parents, not that a parent has the right to a child. Custody was replaced by the idea of parental responsibility and it is now invariable that parents both retain what is called joint parental responsibility. This is intended to reinforce the principle of responsibility rather than rights in relation to children.

A petitioner as a matter of good practice is required to attempt to secure the agreement of the respondent to the proposed arrangements for the children and to get him or her to sign the statement of arrangements. The statement is a lengthy printed form which provides in great detail for the petitioner to set out the residential, educational and care arrangements for each child and deal with the question of how the child is supported.

The practice is problematic. Where a husband and wife are completely at loggerheads it is unlikely that the respondent will sign the statement of arrangements. In the early stages of the new procedure it sometimes happened that a statement of arrangements sent to a respondent or his or her solicitor as a gesture of courtesy prior to the filing of the petition triggered the filing of a petition by the proposed respondent.

FINANCIAL PROVISION FOR THE CHILDREN

The Child Support Act does not give the Child Support Agency jurisdiction to make arrangements for stepchildren, for those in university education, for those over the age of 19, for those who have been married, or those whose parent or parents are habitually resident abroad.

Where a petition is in relation to a second marriage a request for maintenance for stepchildren may be made if the natural father's contribution is small and insufficient and the stepfather has provided a degree of support for the children during the marriage. The breakdown of a second marriage may trigger an application for more maintenance from the natural father; or if the mother has no income of her own or does not receive maintenance and is forced to claim income support, an application will be made by the Child Support Agency for maintenance from the natural father.

The other category of cases in which maintenance can be applied for from the court is where, under Section 8 of the Child Support Act, additional provision is needed in addition to the maximum provided by the formula on which the child support assessment is based, for example where school fees are additionally required or where additional maintenance is required for expenses associated with a child's disability (see Chapter 10).

PROCEDURE

Two copies of the petition have to be taken to a county court which has divorce jurisdiction or to the Principal Registry in London, and a fee of £80 paid for the petition to be issued unless the petitioner is receiving advice under the Green Form scheme. The petition must be accompanied by the marriage certificate, to prove that the parties are married, and two copies of the statement of arrangements. Additionally, if the petitioner is represented by a solicitor and is not receiving assistance to take divorce proceedings under the Green Form scheme, a certificate has to be filed by the solicitor. This states whether or not the solicitor has advised the petitioner in relation to the possibility of reconciliation.

The petitioner has to decide whether the court should serve the petition and other documents by post. If the respondent is unlikely to sign the acknowledgement of service form which accompanies the petition, he or she should be personally served by an enquiry agent. Service cannot be effected by the petitioner. The reason for personal service is that it has to be proved to the court's satisfaction that the existence of the petition and its contents have been brought to the notice of the respondent. The documents which accompany one copy of the petition are a notice of proceedings (which explains that a divorce petition has been filed) and an acknowledgement form (which contains a number of questions for the respondent to answer and which must be returned to the court in 14 days). The respondent has to state where and when the petition was received and indicate whether or not he or she is going to defend the petition or any financial claim in it, as well as whether he or she wishes to be heard on any claim with regard to the children.

Service by an enquiry agent is an additional expense which may be considerable if the respondent wishes to be uncooperative. The agent needs to have a photograph and sufficient description to identify the respondent. After service the agent prepares and swears an affidavit setting out the circumstances in which the respondent was served, the agent having satisfied himself or herself as to the respondent's identity.

If personal service is impossible or if the whereabouts of the respondent are unknown a district judge may make an order providing for substituted service by advertisement in a newspaper if satisfied of the probability that the petition will thus be brought to the respondent's attention. An application for substituted service has to be made by an affidavit filed at court on behalf of the petitioner. Alternatively, if exhaustive enquiries as to the whereabouts of the respondent have failed altogether or if the respondent can be shown to have received the petition, an application should be made for service to be dispensed with. Again, an affidavit setting out the reasons for the application has to be sworn. The district judge may make the order or may require further enquiries to be made before making an actual order.

If a respondent does not have a solicitor he or she will complete the form and sign it. Even if a solicitor does represent the respondent it is for the respondent to sign personally an acknowledgement of service to a petition based on two years' separation, for that signature constitutes consent. The same applies to a petition based on adultery, the signature of the respondent providing the admission. In separation cases, whether based on two years or five years, the respondent should indicate if he or she wishes to be heard on financial matters unless they have already been agreed. The answer given in the acknowledgement of service to the question about financial application is of relevance in these cases because it is possible that the respondent, usually the wife, will want to ensure that if the divorce proceeds it will not be made absolute when the petitioner wants it to be made. The respondent can invite the court to consider her financial circumstances (Section 10, 1973 Matrimonial Causes Act) to ascertain whether they are the best which could be obtained in the circumstances or whether other arrangements should be made. This is a means available in separation-based divorces to delay or, very exceptionally, prevent decree absolute. This is of particular relevance for wives who may lose a possible future widow's pension after a long marriage to a man in well-paid employment. However, the court's powers in relation to pensions is very limited, although the prospective loss of pension has to be taken into account in decisions made by the court on capital (see Chapter 12 and the new Section 25(B) Matrimonial Causes Act 1973 inserted into that Act by the Pensions Act 1995).

Any application for a child to live with a parent with whom they do not already reside has to be the subject of an application for what is called a 'residence order'. Alternatively, where more contact is sought by one parent with the child an application may be made for this under the Children Act. As a preliminary to any formal court process most courts have a conciliation procedure: this requires the applicant to obtain a conciliation appointment before completing a detailed statement in support of his or her claim for residence or contact procedure. Decisions made on this are not in any way connected with the timing of the divorce procedure.

In a case where there is no question of defending a petition – and respondents are usually advised against filing an answer to the allegations in the petition because conduct which is relevant to financial issues can be raised separately in the financial proceedings – the petitioner's next step is to swear what is called an 'affidavit' under the special procedure. The procedure is described thus because it replaces the oral evidence by which a petitioner appeared before a judge in court to 'prove' the contents of his or her petition.

This affidavit consists of a straightforward series of questions to establish the following facts. The petitioner has to confirm that he or she has seen the petition and can amend anything said in it; he or she has to confirm the truth or belief in the truth of its contents. The petitioner also has to say in an adultery case why he or she knows adultery has been committed, and in an unreasonable behaviour case when he or she came to the conclusion that the marriage had broken down. In the latter case the respondent is required to state whether he or she has continued living in the same house and must set out the basis upon which that has happened.

It must always be borne in mind, as explained above, that in cases of unreasonable behaviour and adultery the petitioner cannot suffer the behaviour or the adultery complained of for more than six months without forfeiting the right to complain of them as a basis for divorce.

In cases of separation the affidavit requires information about the addresses occupied by each party since the separation. The affidavit ends with the repetition of the request for a divorce and, if relevant, costs.

A form called a 'Request for Directions' is sent to the court with the affidavit when it has been sworn before a solicitor, who must not be the solicitor representing or advising the petitioner. The court file containing the original petition, the acknowledgement of service and the affidavit is then read by a district judge, who decides whether there is sufficient evidence of breakdown for the marriage to be dissolved. The directions are completed on the same form, with an indication of when the decree is to be pronounced. A decree nisi is pronounced in open court but usually no one attends. At no stage during the divorce process does the petitioner or respondent have to appear at court and at no stage does either party have to explain the arrangements for the children to obtain the court's approval of them.

A divorce is obtained in two stages. First there is a decree nisi pronounced in open court. This is to satisfy the principal requirement of the law in practice that justice shall be seen to be done. This differs from the practice in financial matters or in issues concerning children, which are always held in private. The order made on the pronouncement of the decree nisi recites the date of the marriage, the names of the parties and the names of the children of the family. It refers to the basis of divorce and provides for an order for costs, if relevant. The decree contains a footnote requiring either party taking the child abroad to obtain the consent of the other before doing so and to lodge with the court an undertaking that he or she will return the child within the period stated.

After six complete weeks from the pronouncement of the decree nisi the petitioner can apply on a short form for the decree to be made absolute. This costs £20. There are two circumstances in which it is inadvisable to make the decree absolute at the earliest possible date. The first is if the dissolution of the marriage means that a wife would lose her prospective widow's pension and no compensating arrangement has been taken account of in the negotiations or there is insufficient capital to compensate the wife by giving her more money. The importance of this factor is lessened if there is a potential claim for continuing maintenance.

The other concerns the relatively few cases where one party is the sole owner of the matrimonial home and the other intends to remarry. Remarriage prevents a person who is not the legal owner of the matrimonial home from making a claim for a share of it under the Matrimonial Causes Act 1973 (Section 28(3)). There would still be a residual claim for a proportion of its value but it would be very limited (see Chapter 8). The divorce process is separate from the financial application save for the fact that the intention to make financial claims is stated in the divorce petition. If the petition does not contain any financial claim the petitioner has to apply for leave to make claims before the marriage is dissolved. Where an agreement is reached on financial terms of settlement it may include a division of capital assets which is intended to be the final one. It is usual to ensure that the agreement becomes a consent order. Such an order can only take effect at the same time as or after decree absolute, and where it is agreed in advance of decree absolute it contains the words 'subject to decree absolute'.

It is possible to apply to the court to shortern the time within which the decree can be made absolute. The most usual basis upon which leave will be granted is where a child is expected to be born to either party by a third party and it is intended that the child shall be born legitimate.

Chapter 7

Financial applications

Perhaps partly because a high proportion of marriages break down, many couples postpone the decision to marry, and live together instead. They may never marry. An increasing number of children are born to cohabiting couples and a large body of case law has developed in relation to financial issues which arise on the breakdown of cohabiting arrangements. In some cases couples regulate their relationships by cohabitation contracts.

Cohabitation is outside the remit of this book, but the extent of the social changes it represents has given rise to intensive debate about the differences between cohabitation and marriage. In particular there has been a great deal of public discussion of the merits of marriage contracts, much of it generated by the proposals published by the Law Society's Family Law Committee in 1990. The difficulty in accepting the idea is that it may be said to be against public policy for a married couple to legislate for their financial arrangements during the marriage and provide, as such contracts would, for what would happen on divorce. There is a paradox here because where a widow who has been dependent on her husband makes a claim against his estate (under the Inheritance (Provision for Family and Dependants) Act 1975) if he has left her insufficient to live on, a court considers her claim on the basis of what she might have been awarded if the marriage had ended in divorce instead of death.

It is also ironic that a woman who has cohabited with a man has no claim against him for maintenance for herself when the relationship breaks down, or any claim to a share in his property unless she can establish it by showing what she has contributed to it or what property he has accepted an obligation to give her. Until the Law Reform (Succession) Act 1995 was passed, if she could prove that she had been dependent on him within six months prior to his death she would have a claim against his estate. Now however, under the new Act those eligible to apply for provision out of the estate of anyone who died on or after 1 January 1996 do not have to establish that they were being 'maintained' by the deceased if, during the period of two years ending immediately before the death, they were living in the same household as the deceased as the husband or wife of the deceased. However, the provision is limited to sums required for maintenance. Capital claims can of course be made on behalf of children whether or not their mother was married to their father (Schedule 1 Children Act 1989) and the claim will not necessarily be limited to one claim only.

In 1991 the Law Society asked the government for legislation to recognise marriage contracts as legally enforceable provided the parties had had independent legal advice before signing them, and provided they had amended them when significant changes had occurred, for example if one partner had become disabled or had inherited a large sum of money. The benefit for couples who can adhere to an arrangement made when the future looked rosy would be the saving of the financial costs of breakdown and this perhaps would lighten the emotional trauma.

In the present state of the law any such financial provision agreed in the marriage contract is one of the factors the court takes into account together with all the other factors it is obliged to consider when hearing a financial application by a spouse. Those factors are set out in the Matrimonial Causes Act 1973 (Section 25). A solicitor should provide information about these guidelines at an early point in discussions with the client because they form the framework within which the court decides disputed claims or solicitors help clients settle them. They are:

(a) the income, earning capacity, property and other financial resources which each spouse has or is likely to have in the foreseeable future. The court will also consider whether it would be reasonable to expect either spouse to take steps to increase their earning capacity;
(b) the financial needs, obligations and responsibilities which each spouse has or is likely to have in the foreseeable future;
(c) the standard of living enjoyed by the family before the breakdown of the marriage;

(d) the age of each spouse and the duration of the marriage;
(e) any physical or mental disability of either spouse;
(f) the contributions which each spouse has made to the welfare of the family, including any contribution by looking after the home or caring for the family;
(g) the conduct of each spouse, if that conduct is such that it would in the opinion of the court be inequitable to disregard it. (In practice it is most unusual for the court to decide that a spouse's conduct should affect any financial order that is made);
(h) the value of any benefit which either spouse will lose the chance of acquiring on decree absolute of divorce. The most obvious example is the loss of benefits under the other spouse's pension scheme. There is no exact formula for valuing such possible prospective loss, but even so it is a factor generally taken into account in negotiations and court proceedings.

The court deals at the same time with applications for children who are outside the jurisdiction of the Agency. Where the children are being dealt with by the Agency the level of assessment is another factor the court must consider. In all cases an application for capital may be made to the court; and it is now clearly established, as mentioned above, that more than one application can be made for a child (Schedule 1, Children Act 1989).

In order that a solicitor can advise which claims should be pursued he or she will need to have a summary of the client's income, assets and liabilities. An experienced solicitor may furnish a client with a form to complete before the first interview so that the information can be easily elicited. It is equally important to ascertain the same financial information about the other spouse. Husbands and wives are frequently familiar with each other's circumstances. It is in cases where one or both parties are self-employed that most uncertainty occurs.

It is essential that a client should appreciate two facts about the financial disclosure process, or discovery, as it is called. First, the solicitor has a duty to try to establish the means of the other party. Secondly, in discharging this duty the solicitor has to exercise great care not to seek to enlarge the scope of the work unreasonably. The difficulty is that it is often only when a great deal of costly time has been expended in extracting the information that it becomes apparent that the other party is no longer as wealthy as he or she once was. Conversely, partial disclosure may indicate the existence of hidden assets.

If efforts to reach a settlement have failed it becomes necessary to prepare for a hearing of the application. The steps which must be taken were clearly defined by Mrs Justice Booth in a case decided in 1990 (See Appendix 2). The parties should agree a chronology of the main events in the marriage. This will consist typically of the date of the marriage, the birth of the children, their current status, the occupation of the parties, the date of separation, divorce and relevant information of any other settled relationship. Secondly, the parties should try and agree a list of assets and liabilities. Thirdly, each has to prepare a detailed breakdown of the costs they have incurred to the date of the hearing. What will not be referred to is the substance of Calderbank offers. These are stipulated to be made 'without prejudice save as to costs' (see Chapter 3 and p. 51 below). Correspondence headed thus is to be distinguished from correspondence headed merely 'without prejudice': such correspondence is not open but does not provide protection in relation to costs.

PROCEDURE

If a client is being assisted to obtain a divorce under the Green Form scheme it will not be possible to pursue financial questions until he or she has obtained a legal aid certificate. If a client is paying privately for a divorce he or she may be eligible for legal aid on financial matters. The issuing of a certificate takes several months. In some circumstances where it is necessary to take emergency measures, such as an application to freeze funds or prevent the removal of funds (Chapter 5), it is possible to obtain an emergency certificate, sometimes by telephone.

A client who is not eligible for legal aid or for advice under the Green Form scheme may want advice about financial procedure at the first interview. It may be that the financial conduct of the other party was part of the reason for the marriage breakdown, and if this is so it will be reflected in the petition if the evidence of breakdown is unreasonable behaviour.

Although an application for financial relief can be filed at the same time as the petition the court will only arrange a hearing of it after decree nisi. However, if it is necessary to make an application for interim maintenance, that can be heard at any time after the filing of the divorce petition provided the evidence is available, and subject to the court's timetable. The court's power to vary property rights, to discuss maintenance claims and future claims for capital, and to award capital sums can arise only where there is a decree. If a negotiated settlement seems a possibility it is obviously preferable to defer making an application until negotiations appear to be stalled, because the making of an application may be taken to mean an intention to fight. The progress of negotiations should therefore be kept under constant review.

Most negotiations are conducted in correspondence which is headed 'without prejudice save as to costs' (see Chapter 3 above). This is to protect the correspondence from disclosure, and the sums offered will become known to parties other than the solicitors and their clients only when terms are agreed. It is important to make a reasonable offer or to consider seriously a reasonable offer because there may be serious financial consequences in terms of costs if the case is fought and a lesser sum is awarded than was originally offered. If the other party has rejected a reasonable offer and the amount awarded by the court is less, he or she may also suffer in costs. The protection a without prejudice offer may afford the person offering it is that if it is rejected and the other party does worse in court the other party may be at risk of paying the other spouse's costs from the date the offer was made; although it must always be borne in mind that costs are in the discretion of the court and the without prejudice offers are not made known to the judge until after a judgment has been given and the question of costs is raised. It may be that the justice of the case requires an order for costs against a party who is unable to meet such an order.

There is much to be said for making an open offer in correspondence and also in the affidavit which is filed in support of an application. Where the legal advice is absolutely clear that the offer is a reasonable one, and it is one which the spouse offering it is happy to make, it may be to his or her credit to record it openly.

Lengthy correspondence and exchanges of documents can consume similar costs to a contested court application. A contested application may not be heard for many months or even years. The time between the filing of the application with the first affidavit and the eventual hearing depends on the speed of preparation and filing of affidavits, and the preparedness or ability to provide the necessary documentation and valuations as well as the pressures on the court timetable. Even when it is necessary to proceed with an application to the court, the door to settlement should not be closed. The fact that an application has been made may concentrate the mind of the other party on the issues.

A financial application on behalf of a petitioner pursues the claims set out in the petition. A financial application made on behalf of the respondent makes the claims he or she has stated in the acknowledgement of service will be pursued. It is vital that the claim for a wife should include periodical payments (unless she expressly, in writing, instructs the solicitor not to do so), lump sum and property adjustment. The exclusion of the last in a leading bankruptcy case involved a subsequent negligence action against the solicitors (*Re Gorman* 1990 All ER 717).

Usually the property adjustment order sought is in respect of the matrimonial home, which must be accurately described with its Land Registry number if it is registered land; details of the mortgagees are required and the rule that mortgagees must be served with a copy of the notice must be complied with. The notice of application is in Form M11 or M13 (see Appendix 5, p. 176).

In the affidavit in support of the application the petitioner sets out the financial history of the marriage. In a long marriage it will not be necessary to recite the details of every home purchased and sold but the court requires sufficient information to be able to form an opinion based on facts which are relevant to financial matters. The frugality or spendthrift nature of either party should be referred to in the document but the presentation of a case is not enhanced by dwelling on conduct that has had no financial repercussions.

The court's concern is with matters relevant to the guidelines in the legislation. Thus it will be appropriate to mention loss of work through sickness: this may affect earning capacity. It will also be relevant that one party habitually gambled so that the standard of living may not have reflected the true financial potential of the couple. Whether or not certain facts should be included or omitted, glossed over or emphasised, is a matter of judgement, and a petitioner or respondent acting for himself or herself with assistance from a solicitor will require help at this important juncture when the contents of the affidavit are finally considered before being sworn and placed on the court file.

Because the affidavits contain the evidence on which the contested issues will be determined it is vital that nothing of financial importance should be overlooked. At the hearing each party will give oral evidence so that the other or his or her solicitor can cross-examine him to test the evidence, but fresh evidence cannot be raised at the hearing unless it relates to a very recent development.

The solicitor who filed the financial application and affidavit in support should at an early stage seek the agreement of his or her opponent on the directions which should be given by the court. In other words, solicitors are under a duty to try and agree what evidence should be provided to enable the court to make a decision. It is provided in the Family Proceedings Rules of 1991 as amended that when one party has sworn an affidavit it should be served on the other or his or her solicitors and answered 14 days after receipt. This rule is not strictly observed: it may be impracticable to expect the other party to obtain the necessary documentation to prepare an affidavit in reply, and the other party may be waiting the outcome of a legal aid application. A longer period of time can be agreed. The process of applying for legal aid may be a tactic adopted by one party to delay matters and it is particularly irksome to the other party, whose financial circumstances appear to make him or her equally eligible for legal aid but who has been advised that his or her financial circumstances clearly rule out eligibility.

Courts differ in how they ensure that the Practice Direction (see Appendix 2) is complied with. Some courts actually prescribe themselves the further steps to be taken before trial in their own orders for directions. Other courts leave to practitioners the responsibility for deciding upon the steps to be taken. In a straightforward case, directions orders state the time within which affidavits will be sworn and provide an opportunity for a further affidavit by the applicant. They will then go on to provide for discovery (the disclosure of financial information).

Where solicitors agree on an order for directions, the solicitor applying for the order obtains the written agreement of the other in a summons which sets out the terms that have been agreed. Where delays in providing information can be anticipated, because it will involve correspondence with banks or accountants or because there are foreign assets, the directions should provide for an appropriate period within which further evidence should be obtained. In a straightforward case where no affidavit has been sworn by the respondent, the order will provide for it and perhaps for the applicant to have the right of reply if necessary. It may be provided that there shall be no further affidavits so an application to a district judge can always be made for leave to file one if relevant. The order will usually provide for a questionnaire to be served by each party to establish the means and resources of the other party to the extent that they have not been provided by the affidavits. The provision of documentary evidence in support of the replies to the questionnaire will also be necessary. A time limit is set for the replies.

Where there are assets such as a matrimonial home a direction is usually made for a valuation if values cannot be agreed. The parties may agree that there should be a valuation by a jointly appointed valuer or, if they are unable to agree that, each should be able to call his or her own valuer. Such evidence is usually limited to one valuer each. The client and solicitor have to weigh very carefully the risks of calling a valuer to give evidence at the hearing. It may be necessary if the other valuation is much lower or higher than expected and an agreed figure is impossible to arrive at. It will certainly be more expensive, and in legally aided cases the cost of a valuation has to be authorised in advance by the Legal Aid Board before the valuer can be instructed.

The most valuable asset in a middle-aged marriage may be the pension or pension entitlement which one party has. Although the loss of a prospective widow's or widower's pension is a factor which the court is obliged to consider it has no power to split a pension, and the transfer value of a pension fund is an important item in a clean-break case where no continuing maintenance is likely to be awarded (see Chapter 12). The Pensions Act (see Introduction, p. 5) introduced into the Matrimonial Causes Act 1973 a new Section 25(B). This imposes a duty on the court to examine the pensions provision and gives the court power to impose an attachment order on the trustees of the fund when the pension becomes payable. It is likely to mean that there will be fewer clean breaks in future but the way in which the new section will be applied will depend upon regulations the government has yet to make.

Other assets whose value will be sought are stocks and shares and building society funds. These need to be updated at the time of the hearing. Where one party earns his or her living from a family company its worth will not be an asset to be divided, particularly if it produces the income which will continue to support the family, but some idea of its value is necessary if one party is to retain it.

There have been a number of court decisions, notably *B* v. *B* (1989 1 FLR 119) in which the judgment of the court made it plain that expensive accountants' costs of a company valuation, or in this case a professional practice, were unnecessary.

Complex questions may arise in relation to liabilities, for example loans to a company which are secured by a charge on the matrimonial home and which may be repayable before any sale or transfer of it could take place. Documentary evidence of loans will be necessary.

Where the discovery process does not result in the production of documents which may be relevant to establish the means of a party there is provision (1991 2 FLR 62) to apply for a production appointment. If an order is made (and it can be made against a third party such as a bank or employer) the party against whom it is made has to attend the production appointment with the relevant documents. The purpose of the rule is to save some of the costs of lengthening the eventual ancillary relief hearing, and of course to facilitate preparation for it.

The remaining terms of an order for directions will usually include provision that the case shall be heard with each party giving oral evidence when certificates of readiness are provided and a date has been fixed for the hearing. In some county courts the final hearing where the case is not estimated to take more than perhaps half a day is conducted by a solicitor. In other cases it may be more economical for a barrister to be instructed. This is usually the case in the London area. If a barrister represents a client a representative from the firm of solicitors must be present to take a full note. A busy solicitor who does little advocacy but spends his or her working time negotiating and drafting documents may prefer to brief a barrister whose experience in appearing before district and county court judges and High Court judges is more extensive. This division of labour and responsibility is often criticised as being more expensive. There are arguments on both sides.

In London experienced solicitors nearly always have higher staff and office overheads than a barrister, so the solicitor's hourly rate may be higher than that of the barrister, whose overheads may be lower but who spends most of his or her time in advocacy in the courts and preparation for trials. An argument against this practice is that the solicitor's clerk who takes a note of the hearing is an additional cost, as is the time spent by the solicitor preparing the documentation for counsel and going to one or more conferences with counsel in preparation for the hearing. A client represented by one solicitor practitioner at a hearing when the spouse was represented by a solicitor and a barrister later commented, 'You had to do everything but she had one to watch and listen and one to think.'

In a case where very complex questions of law are involved it may be considered that the matter should be placed for hearing before a High Court judge. If this is not agreed by both sides the decision of the district judge on the matter will be final unless either party decides to appeal.

The question of instructing counsel often does not arise until it becomes apparent that attempts to settle have failed and the application has then to be heard by the court. It may be anticipated that the case will require a barrister for advice at an earlier stage where there is concern about which strategy should be adopted. For example, the husband in the case of a short marriage where the wife was formerly a high earner but now has two very young children may be concerned to have a settlement on the basis that provision for the wife will be capital only, and perhaps more than half of that will be represented by the matrimonial home so that the children will have continuity of home and the wife the security of knowing that she will not have to sell. The wife may take the view that resumption of her career will be a problem and that she will need to seek maintenance. If a compromise offering some maintenance limited in time to two or three years is unacceptable it will be apparent that a trial of the issues is inevitable.

The issues of capital and maintenance are inextricably involved and their resolution may be affected just as much by external factors such as the condition of the housing market, the availability of alternative housing, and the level of interest rates as by the abilities of the parties and their representatives to compromise.

Despite the growth of part-time work for women many will still require maintenance for an indefinite period. There are two categories where it is unlikely that these claims will be pursued or where they will be left dormant: where the husband, and possibly the wife, is unemployed or where the wife has never been dependent or taken a career break which has affected her earning capacity. Where the wife is wholly or partly dependent she can negotiate dismissal of her maintenance claims if the capital provided is sufficient to give her not only a home but investment income. Such provision is unlikely except in the case of significantly better off families.

The Matrimonial and Family Proceedings Act of 1984 recognised that the objective of the 1973 Matrimonial Causes Act to keep the parties in the position they would have been if the marriage had not broken down was wholly unrealistic. For all but the most wealthy, divorce is an impoverishing process to some degree. Remarriage may change the circumstances of divorced men and women but it is expected that two in three second marriages will break down and many divorced people prefer to rebuild their lives first on their own. Of great importance to wives needing maintenance is the knowledge that if they cohabit or remarry, their former husband will be entitled usually to the discharge of their maintenance order, and unless the second relationship breaks down they will be unlikely to revive maintenance claims against their first husband.

The solicitor's task is to help clients decide what they and their families need and whether those needs can be met from the resources available. If the only assets are a mortgaged house, a car and an insurance policy with little value, the outcome of negotiations will depend on what can be afforded. If the mortgage is low and the wife is working full time with school-aged children, she may be able to take on the mortgage if the mortgagees agree. She may not be able to increase the mortgage to buy her husband's share of the equity. On the other hand she may be able to take on the mortgage subject to her husband or another salary earner guaranteeing its payment, particularly if she will be dependent upon maintenance for some of the payment.

If the husband remains joint owner of the house he will continue to be responsible for the mortgage with his wife and will be restricted in his opportunity to buy a house for himself unless he forms another relationship. If he succeeds in buying a home while remaining owner of the first one he may be liable to capital gains tax on the proportion he has retained when his former wife eventually sells.

From the early 1980s the clean break in relation to capital and maintenance grew in popularity. A husband often transferred his share of equity to his wife. The money it represented enabled her to remain in the matrimonial home and, provided she was able to pay the mortgage, or if out of work received housing benefit, the family remained housed. In many cases nominal maintenance was awarded for children because children's maintenance claims cannot be dismissed. Such an outcome is now exceedingly problematic. If a wife now or in the future is unemployed with dependent children the Child Support Agency has the power to seek provision for the children from the former husband. The existence of the clean break is no barrier, however much equity it represents, although as a result of recent changes in the regulations the formula for assessing support is modified where a transfer has been for the benefit of the children.

In cases where the maintenance of children is not a complicating factor, for example where they may have ceased full-time education, the solution of a clean break is not necessarily the most satisfactory one. Divorcing couples may be very anxious to have no continuing financial ties but dismissal of maintenance may not be prudent even if a generous capital settlement with a clean break is possible. Economic uncertainty about the future means that no solicitor, however able, can be sure that either a clean break or continuing maintenance is safe. The clean break will seem to have been a wise decision to a wife whose husband later becomes unemployed. On the other hand, if the husband later obtains far more lucrative employment which might have warranted higher maintenance than that which formed the basis of the capital sum paid for a clean break, it will appear unfortunate. The new Section 25(B) of the Matrimonial Causes Act 1973 will further complicate the issue. From the husband's point of view the early remarriage of his ex-wife may make a generous clean break seem wasted; but it could only be set aside if the former wife intended at the time of the settlement to remarry or concealed her intention to do so by failing to declare it in answer to the question about remarriage on the financial statement both parties have to complete for filing at the court.

Since the 1984 Act the court has had the power to dismiss wives' maintenance rights or provide for their dismissal after a period of time such as three or four years. Dismissal of rights to maintenance is invariably accompanied by a dismissal of the right to claim against the estate of the spouse after death (Inheritance (Provision for Family and Dependants) Act 1975).

Where continuing maintenance is agreed or ordered by the court it can later be dismissed if circumstances change: the wife may obtain full-time well-paid employment or receive a substantial inheritance so that her circumstances improve sufficiently to justify dismissal of her claim. In the usual course of events either party will seek to vary maintenance from time to time as circumstances change or inflation increases. Some couples provide in their agreed order a formula linking future increases to the Retail Price Index. This provides very low increases in times of low inflation and is not appropriate if the financial circumstances of either party are likely to change substantially.

There are three other critical factors which influence negotiation. First, orders or settlements in relation to capital are final. Only in extreme cases (such as the immediate death of the members of the family who are to benefit: *Barder* v. *Barder and Caluori*) can they be set aside. If it transpired that there was a failure to disclose an asset or source of income which would have affected the outcome, or if there was a failure to disclose an intention to marry, an application to set aside an application might succeed. It might also succeed if an asset whose value was concealed is sold for a much higher figure than was used in the calculation of the overall assets so that the whole basis for the division could be shown to have been false.

Secondly, costs, as noted before, are a reason for avoiding or limiting litigation. But where no agreement has been possible because the full financial picture is not clear or because one party or both cannot compromise on the figures, the costs may have increased to a level where their payment becomes another issue in dispute. Costs can make a vital difference to the amount of capital available for the family to live on. The strict rules now governing preparation for a case were laid down after a trial in which costs were disproportionate to the assets involved (see Appendix 2).

Concern to reduce costs is one of the principal reasons for the government's consultation paper *Mediation and the Grounds for Divorce* (Cmnd 2799). It is also the reason why many courts have adopted the procedure of reviewing a case with all the parties at a point when a settlement may be possible.

The third factor is time, which is closely related to the question of costs. While a case is being litigated in court and negotiations continue over attempts to settle claims, events may occur in the parties' lives which change the basis on which the claims are made. An accident may render a breadwinner unable to work but he or she may be awarded a capital settlement if there is a question of someone else being responsible for the accident. One party may be offered employment abroad and a decision has to be made. Inheritance may enlarge the assets which have to be divided. Care arrangements for a rich parent of one party may consume the capital he or she is expected to inherit so that it ceases to be a possible resource to which the court might have had regard. A woman may form a relationship and wish to remarry. A cohabiting woman's relationship may break down so that her husband may be liable for maintenance when he had expected to have no further responsibility. Costs increase with the time taken to determine the outcome of a claim, but since the final capital settlement cannot be reviewed except as explained above the intervention of fate in a fundamental way before a hearing inevitably causes a reassessment of the overall situation.

Chapter 8

Insolvency

Marriage breakdown causes debts to be incurred but is sometimes the result of problems arising from an accumulation of unmanageable debt. If one spouse is made bankrupt his or her property passes to or vests in the person appointed to be the trustee in bankruptcy when the bankruptcy order is made.

Although insolvency giving rise to bankruptcy is now decreasing, the number of bankruptcies between 1988 and 1992 increased from 7,717 to 32,106. Where one or both parties to a marriage are involved in small businesses with debt difficulties they will need specialist advice if they are to negotiate the pitfalls of possible bankruptcy.

The law on bankruptcy is now contained in the Insolvency Act 1986 and the Insolvency Rules of the same year.

If there is a possibility of one spouse becoming bankrupt the solicitor acting for the other will want to make a bankruptcy search to ascertain whether a bankruptcy order has already been made. This simple procedure involves a bankruptcy search at the Land Charges Department in Plymouth (see p. 223). There is a fee of £1, or £2 by telephone. If the result is PA (B) it means that a bankruptcy petition has been presented or if the result is WO (B) a bankruptcy order has been made. If the property is registered an application must be made to HM Land Registry with the title number of the property quoted in the application for office copies of the entries on the register. For example, if the property is in the name of one spouse, and a bankruptcy petition has been presented, the register may show a 'creditors' notice', or if a bankruptcy order has actually been made it will show 'bankruptcy inhibition'. If a property is jointly owned a caution will have been registered by the trustee in bankruptcy.

A debtor who is unable to pay his or her debts can present a petition. The petition must list his or her creditors, secured and unsecured, the assets, and the dependants, and must list any outstanding distress or other proceedings as well as the possibility of an individual voluntary arrangement (IVA).

The effect of possible bankruptcy on the home is serious. A landlord can levy distress for three months' rent. A lease can be forfeited. Where there is a bankruptcy order the trustee in bankruptcy who represents the creditors will want to realise the bankrupt's interests in order to pay the creditors. It is important to emphasise that a debtor owing more than £750 on unsecured debts is at risk of a bankruptcy petition and if a petition is filed in respect of such a debt or payments due under it the bankruptcy will relate to the whole of the debt.

A creditor may decide not to take the alternative step available, which is to sue for a debt, but instead to present a statutory demand. The creditor does this where he or she considers there to be a risk of the debtor's property being reduced in the three-month period within which a bankruptcy petition must be filed. In bankruptcy the bankrupt is left with the tools of his trade and household possessions unless the latter include valuable items such as a motor car which can be sold. The bankrupt will be left with income to meet the needs of himself or herself and family, and any order for maintenance made during bankruptcy proceedings will be stayed until the bankruptcy has been discharged.

The bankruptcy continues until discharge, when the bankrupt is released from all bankruptcy debts and restrictions with some exceptions, which include family or domestic awards. There is some doubt about the effect of the Insolvency Act on the position since 1986. Formerly, arrears of maintenance could not be recovered but a lump sum could and a leading case in 1969 resulted in annual maintenance of £3,000 being capitalised as a lump sum of £33,600 which was ordered to be paid by the bankrupt. The position is, however, no longer clear-cut. Specialist advice should be taken before a decision is made as to the course to be adopted.

The greatest disadvantage of bankruptcy is the loss of the bankrupt's home. An alternative is an individual voluntary arrangement. Under such arrangement, if the creditors as a class agree, an insolvency practitioner is instructed. A key question in making a decision about this course is whether there will be sufficient assets to pay the creditors and the fees of the insolvency practitioner. One advantage is that the heavy fees of bankruptcy, averaging about 60 per cent of the assets, can be avoided so that there is more money available to pay the creditors. Between 1988 and 1992 there was a sixfold increase in the number of IVAs. Other alternatives which are outside the ambit of this book include an administration order, a restriction order or a deed of arrangement.

This part of the chapter will consider the effect of the possibility of bankruptcy on the transfer of the matrimonial home, and the effect of a transfer after bankruptcy. First, although bankruptcy does not immediately affect sales or transfers of the ownership of a matrimonial home which have already been completed, Section 39 of the Matrimonial Causes Act 1973 provides that the Bankruptcy Court can set aside any property transfer order in matrimonial proceedings. Under the Insolvency Act of 1986 a trustee in bankruptcy can use Section 423, 340 or 339 to set aside a transfer. Under the first section the trustee has to show an intention on the part of the bankrupt to defeat the interests of the trustee. There is no time limit in which this step must be taken. However, if the property has been transferred to someone who has no knowledge of the bankruptcy the transaction will not be set aside.

A trustee in bankruptcy can make an application under Section 340 of the Insolvency Act and the court will make an order setting aside the transfer if it is satisfied that the result has been to put one of the creditors in a better position than would otherwise have been the case. If the transaction was at an under-value, the trustee can make an application to set it aside within five years of the transaction. If the transaction was not at an under-value but an associate of the bankrupt was put in a better position as a result of the transfer, the application to set the transfer aside can be made within two years. If preference was not given to an associate of the bankrupt, the trustee can make an application within six months of the transfer. In each case the trustee has to show that the bankrupt was insolvent or became insolvent as a result of the transfer.

The third provision enabling a trustee to apply for a transfer to be set aside is under Section 339. A transaction under this section can be set aside if it is at an under-value and it must have taken place within five years prior to the date when the bankruptcy petition was presented. It can be set aside within two years if it can be shown that the bankrupt is not already insolvent or did not become insolvent as a result of transfer. When the application is made after the two-year period it will be for the bankrupt's spouse to show that the bankrupt did not become bankrupt as a result of the transfer.

In a leading case on the right of a trustee in bankruptcy to set aside a transfer to a wife prior to a bankruptcy it was argued that Section 24 of the Matrimonial Causes Act was there to protect a wife but not to defeat a trustee in bankruptcy. In that case however (*Re Abbott* 1983 1 Ch 45), the trustee did not succeed in setting aside the transfer but it was emphasised that each case must be looked at in the light of its own particular circumstances'.

In a later case (*Re Kumar* 1993 1 WLR 224) the wife argued that she had paid sufficient for the transfer because she had given up other claims for capital and the transfer of the house should not be considered to have been at an under-value. She failed in this argument because she had accepted responsibility for a mortgage of £30,000 on the house in question and it had a net equity in excess of £100,000, that is to say it was worth more than £100,000 after account was taken of the mortgage of £30,000 so she had not actually 'paid' for what she claimed she should have.

It is possible to put forward arguments against an application to set aside a transfer. It is worth noting that the trustee probably cannot apply for a sale of property under the Law of Property Act 1925 until the court has made an order in his or her favour under the Insolvency Act.

The effect of the three provisions above is to allow a trustee to set aside a transfer if he or she can show that the spouse has unfairly benefited from the transaction. The spouse can still argue the extent of his or her beneficial interest and this is the most vital question in proceedings where the possibility of bankruptcy exists.

The questions that need to be considered will be questions of tactics in relation to whether or not the trustee in bankruptcy should be given an opportunity to value property which will be included in a bankruptcy order; if the trustee does not have access to the property he or she may not appreciate its full worth.

In a recent leading case where a husband by consent transferred the matrimonial home to his wife (an order being made in the county court to that effect) a bankruptcy order was made against the husband six days later. The trustee in bankruptcy was later able to obtain a declaration from the court that the terms of the order providing for the transfer of the home were void against him (Section 284 of the Insolvency Act 1986). The result was that the home was held by the wife and the trustee in bankruptcy in equal shares. The court has to consider what is just and fair in all the circumstances, having regard to good faith and honest intention. If, between the presentation of a bankruptcy petition and the making of a bankruptcy order, a potential bankrupt wishes to dispose of property for the benefit of creditors this can be approved by the court, and would be the case where a purchaser had been found for the home at market value. In the case referred to (*re Fling* 1993 FLR 210) the court had information about the financial background and the parties knew of the impending risk of bankruptcy.

When a bankruptcy order has been made the bankrupt's assets form part of his or her estate in the bankruptcy so that the Family Court cannot make an order for ancillary relief and the only possibility open to the bankrupt's spouse is to try to annul the bankruptcy. The wife in the case of *Re Holiday* (1981 Ch 405) took this step. She had been granted a decree nisi in 1975 and in early March 1976 filed a notice of her intention to proceed with her application for ancillary relief. The husband filed his own petition for bankruptcy on the day when the mortgage instalments were in arrears and his liabilities exceeded his assets. The husband's trustee in bankruptcy applied for a sale of the matrimonial home and the wife made a cross-application to annul the bankruptcy. The trustee in bankruptcy succeeded. The wife's appeal failed even though the court considered that it was possible that the husband's motive for petitioning in bankruptcy was to defeat his wife's claim for a transfer of property order.

The time when a bankrupt's assets became part of his estate was the decisive factor in the case of *Re Dennis* (A Bankrupt) 1995 2 FLR 387. The husband and wife owned two properties as joint tenants. On 21 September 1982 the husband committed an act of bankruptcy by failing to comply with a bankruptcy notice. On 20 December 1982 a bankruptcy petition was presented. On 24 February 1983 the wife died, leaving her property to the two children of the marriage. On 11 November 1983 the husband was adjudged bankrupt. The trustee in bankruptcy sought a declaration that all the property which included the wife's entitlement was subject to the bankruptcy. The High Court decided that the property became that of the trustee in bankruptcy when the husband had been adjudicated bankrupt. The husband had inherited the wife's property because the survivor of joint property inherits it. He had become bankrupt after the wife's death. It was common ground that the husband's bankruptcy severed or broke the joint tenancy so that the properties became owned by each of them, the husband and the wife as tenants in common in equal shares. The question the court had to decide was whether the tenancy was severed by the husband's act of bankruptcy on 21 September 1982 or later, when he was adjudicated bankrupt on 11 November 1983 after the wife's death. The Court of Appeal decided in favour of the wife's personal representatives that the bankruptcy related back to the first act of bankruptcy and its effect was that the joint tenancy in the properties was severed at that date so that the deceased wife's share of the properties did not belong to the trustee in bankruptcy but to her children. The trustee in bankruptcy could only take the husband's share.

The spouse of a bankrupt will be concerned to obtain the help of a solicitor in dealing with the trustee in bankruptcy. He or she will be advised that the trustee in bankruptcy is in a very strong legal position but it may be possible to negotiate with him or her. The trustee needs to know who lives in the home and who has contributed to it and what the spouse claims his or her interests to be. The trustee will want to know whether agreement can be obtained to a valuation of the property and whether there is any possibility of the spouse purchasing the trustee in bankrupt's interest, that is to say the interest of the bankrupt.

The trustee will also be concerned to establish the extent of any mortgage debt and whether the mortgagee intends to bring possession proceedings, as well as the insurance arrangements and whether there exists any endowment policy and in whose name it is. The principal concern of the spouse will be to ensure that the solicitor makes the trustee realise that notwithstanding the co-operation given to the trustee there may be an arguable case against the sale of the home.

The Bankruptcy Court has the power to order the sale of the home on the application by the trustee under Section 336 of the Insolvency Act. The trustee can apply under Section 336 of the Insolvency Act for power to terminate or suspend the right of occupation of a spouse under Section 1 of the Matrimonial Homes Act 1983. This Act applies when the house is in the name of the bankrupt alone. Alternatively, if there is no question of a spouse's right of occupation the trustee can apply for an order for sale of the property under Section 30 of the Law of Property Act 1925 because under that section 'any person interested', which includes a trustee in bankruptcy, can apply to the court for such an order

The power applies only to property which is not a matrimonial home. However, the trustee in bankruptcy has to obtain formal sanction from the Creditors' Committee or from the Official Receiver to take such proceedings and the solicitor acting for the spouse may be able to ensure that there are problems in the way of a sale in the hope of forcing the trustee in bankruptcy to think again about the application.

In considering one of the above applications the court is obliged to consider, apart from the interest of the creditors, the conduct of a spouse or former spouse if it contributed to the bankruptcy, the needs and financial resources of the spouse or former spouse and the needs of any children. A cohabitee is not protected by having his or her rights considered under the Insolvency Act in the same way.

Obviously, the interests of creditors outweigh all the others. Exceptional circumstances may prevail to prevent a sale, for example if the postponement of the payment of debts would not cause great hardship to the creditors, or where the house has been adapted for a handicapped person, where a spouse is terminally ill or when emigration is a possibility.

Where a home is not solely owned by the bankrupt there is a period of 12 months in which the house can be sold or the bankrupt's interest bought out, but this must take place with the approval of the trustee in bankruptcy. There is a further option of a charge on the house by the trustee if a sale is unlikely.

Because the law limits the ability of a spouse to prevent a sale it is important to establish the extent of his or her interest in a property owned or partly owned by a bankrupt. Where the house is solely owned by the bankrupt there are the following possibilities.

Section 17 of the Married Women's Property Act 1882 can be used to establish a share of ownership. Section 37 of the Matrimonial Proceedings and Property Act 1970 provides that contributions in money or money's worth to the improvements may be proved to enlarge the share claimed by the spouse under Section 17 or an application made to the county court or the Family Division of the High Court can result in a sale being ordered or postponed. If the property is owned jointly under Section 39 of the Matrimonial Proceedings and Property Act 1970 the spouse's interest can be proved provided the application is made within three years of the dissolution or annulment of the marriage. Alternatively, if the house is owned jointly and the marriage was dissolved or annulled more than three years before, or if a third party is an owner, Section 30 of the Law of Property Act can be used. Section 24 of the Matrimonial Causes Act is unavailable to the bankrupt's spouse unless the bankruptcy order has not yet been made.

Where a house is jointly owned by a bankrupt and his or her spouse, the tendency of the trustee in bankruptcy may be to regard the joint ownership as depriving the creditors of half the equity in the house because the whole of the property may have been purchased by the bankrupt. The situation may of course be the reverse, namely that the bankrupt's spouse has paid for the whole of the property but that it has been bought in joint names. Where there is joint ownership the trustee in bankruptcy has to establish the joint beneficial or equitable entitlement, that is to say the proportion to which each spouse will be entitled on the basis of the contribution made to the property's acquisition.

The document transferring the ownership will be a transfer in the case of registered land or a conveyance in the case of unregistered land. Where a property has been conveyed into joint names it should be conclusive evidence that the parties intended to hold the property in equal shares unless fraud or mistake can be proved, as would be the case where a bankrupt and a spouse purchased a property after a bankruptcy order. If in such circumstances it can be shown that the intention was to put the property in the spouse's sole name and the family should not face eviction the point may be conceded by the trustee. It all depends on the circumstances.

The vital question is the wording which has been used to establish in the transfer or conveyance how the husband and wife intended to share the property. As will be explained in Chapter 9, where the parties acquire a property jointly, they hold it on the basis of a joint tenancy, which means that the survivor will inherit the whole property unless a restriction is placed on the title to the effect that one survivor cannot alone give title to the property. Such a restriction indicates the existence of a tenancy in common. The property may be purchased on a tenancy in common basis, with a declaration of trust which may set out the intention of the parties that the property should be owned in equal shares or in unequal shares. If the parties separate, one may serve a notice of severance of the joint tenancy in order to create a tenancy in common (see Appendix 1). That does not of itself establish that the parties intend that the property shall be shared equally but it enables either party thereafter to leave his or her share by will. So far as bankruptcy is concerned the matter does not end there.

In a 1986 case (*Goodman* v. *Gallant* 1 FLR 513) some years after the breakdown of a marriage in which the husband had purchased the matrimonial home on a mortgage in his sole name he subsequently conveyed the property jointly to the wife and her boyfriend. The wording in the conveyance, the transfer document, stated that the property was conveyed to them on a trust for sale and to hold the net proceeds of sale upon trust for themselves as joint tenants. Subsequently, the wife severed the joint tenancy, in a notice which said that the property would then belong to her and the boyfriend in equal shares. She later claimed that they did not own it equally. In an action for a declaration on the matter the Court of Appeal held that the words in the conveyance were comprehensive unless the document was set aside or rectified. In other words, both parties were held to have an equal interest.

In a case involving bankruptcy (*re Gorman* 1990 AE 717) the circumstances were complicated by the failure of the wife's solicitors to apply for property adjustment when she obtained a divorce. They applied for ancillary relief but in relation only to maintenance for the husband to pay to the wife and for provision for the mortgage instalments. Four years later, in 1982, the husband was made bankrupt and before that happened the wife paid the mortgage arrears in order to avoid a possession order. She continued to pay the mortgage instalments and spent approximately £7,000 on improvements. Seven years later, when the debts amounted to £150,000 and the equity in the house was worth £100,000, the trustee applied for a sale. The result was that an order for sale was deferred so that the wife had an option to purchase the trustee in bankruptcy's shares in certain events.

What emerges from the decided cases is that it is not only the wording of the document of transfer of the conveyance that is most important, but also the wording of the legal charge or mortgage. It is clear that if there is no restriction, that is to say no tenancy in common, it does not mean that the owners own the property equally. However, the severance of the tenancy does not mean that equality is created and it may be the case that the parties will receive proportions equivalent to their contribution.

If the wording of the document is not clear the court will be concerned to establish whether there is a binding obligation or implied trust to define the interest of the owners. In a case where one party provides the purchase money and it is held in the name of the other there will be a resulting trust. There will be a constructive trust if there has been a declared intention to share the interest or there is evidence of a clear agreement. These trusts or obligations arise from the time of the agreement.

To establish entitlement to a share of ownership in a property held in another's name a claimant has to show that there was a common intention to share the interest and that he or she has subsequently acted to his or her disadvantage, or detriment as lawyers describe it. The proof of common intention may be evidenced by mortgage payments or household expenses: the contributions may be considered corroborative evidence of the intention to share and they may quantify the extent of the entitlement or beneficial interest. The court may infer that there is a resulting or implied trust even if there is no evidence in writing if someone living in a property has spent money on it as he or she would be unlikely to do if there was no question of sharing ownership..

The position of a cohabitee is not necessarily the same as that of a spouse but the distinction has not always been made, as in the recent case of *Lloyds Bank plc* v. *Rossett* 1990 1 All ER 1111.

Many of the leading cases where there has been a dispute about the extent of a party's beneficial interest are cases of cohabitees where courts could not exercise their discretion to vary property rights under Section 24 of the Matrimonial Causes Act; but they underlined the fact that the courts' concern is with evidence of common intention; they often find a resulting trust to the effect that the contributions to the acquisition of the property give rise to a right to a proportionate share.

Factors which may be important include the value of a discount, as in the purchase of a council flat. However, the party who has acquired the discount will not obtain credit for it if there is clear evidence that the ownership of the flat was transferred into joint names on the basis that the party should share it equally even if there was no express indication by way of a declaration of the transfer showing how the interests were to be shared. This was the basis on which in the case of *Savill* v. *Goodall* 1993 FLR 755 the Court of Appeal did not allow the appeal of a girlfriend that her share of the interest should take account of the discount. The discount in that case had been 42 per cent and the parties took into account the period of 12 years prior to the transfer when the girlfriend's former husband became a tenant with 100 per cent mortgage. The girlfriend and boyfriend paid monthly instalments of mortgage for a year after the transfer, which took place in 1984, the boyfriend having lived in the property since 1977. The court considered that the agreement or understanding reached by the parties that the house was to be owned jointly in equal shares was not affected by their contributions. Because it had been agreed that the boyfriend would pay the mortgage, his share was to be debited with the amount of the principal owing on the mortgage and the costs of redeeming it. The girlfriend conceded that her payments of the mortgage after the separation would be considered to be an occupation rent, and before the proceeds of sale could be divided between them, account would be taken of those liabilities.

The adjustments made by the court when the trustee in bankruptcy seeks a declaration of the interests of the parties in a property was shown in the case of re *Pavlou* (1993 WLR 1046). Here the husband and wife owned the matrimonial home on a joint tenancy basis. The husband left in January 1983. The wife remained, and paid the instalments of capital and interest on the mortgage, and also spent money on repairs and improvements. Three and a half years later she obtained a decree nisi and eight months later, in March 1987, the husband was made bankrupt. The effect of the bankruptcy order severed the tenancy so that the property became owned by them in equal shares. The court ordered a sale but provided for allowance to be made for the wife's expenditure on the property before and after the bankruptcy so far as it resulted in an increase in value, so she would be entitled against the trustee in bankruptcy to credit for one half of the amount spent on repairs and improvements, one half of the amount calculated in relation to the increased value of the property and one half of the capital element in the payment of the mortgage instalments. It was also held that the wife should pay an occupation rent from the date of her divorce petition but an allowance for the mortgage interest payments since the date the husband had left would be set against it. As it was put in another decision in a cohabitation case (*Bernard* v. *Josephs* 1982 3 ER 162): 'If the woman has left she is entitled to receive an occupation rent but if the man has kept up all the mortgage repayments he is entitled to credit for her share of the payments.'

It cannot be too strongly emphasised that in the absence of evidence of a common intention the carrying out of work by the non-earning spouse is insufficient to establish agreement. The cases where a sole bankrupt owner's spouse (or cohabitee) has been successful in establishing a beneficial or enforceable interest are exceptions rather than the rule. The trustee in bankruptcy prefers the certainty of a jointly owned property with equal shares where the proportion which will be available on sale to distribute among the creditors is known, to one where the beneficial interest of the non-bankrupt spouse is not defined and may be established only by laborious proceedings. It should again be stressed that the courts have a different approach in those cases where couples have not been married and those where they have divorced. It was expressed by the judge in the case of *Hammond* v. *Mitchell* to be the difference between, in the case of formerly married couples, 'a forward looking perspective' and, in the case of the unmarried, 'a painfully detailed retrospect' involving detailed accounting of contributions and payments.

Further complications arise in cases where the home is owned by a third party such as a partnership or a company.

The Bankruptcy Court takes into account the interests of the family against the creditors. In matrimonial proceedings, in contrast, the children are the paramount interest the courts consider. The case of *Mullard* v. *Mullard*, however, established that if there are debts but no bankruptcy it would not be right to prefer the claims of creditors to those of the children since in that case the powers of the court under the Matrimonial Causes Act were being exercised.

Section 337 of the Insolvency Act 1986 provides some minimal protection for children by ensuring that if the bankrupt has some interest in the home and if children under 18 are living with him or her, the bankrupt has the right not to be evicted or excluded except by court order. An occupation is a charge on the bankrupt's estate which is now vested in the trustee in bankruptcy. On the trustee's application to the court, the court will consider the interests described above, which it is obliged to consider under Section 336 (4) of the Act. The most that can be expected for the family is a postponement of the sale. In the case of *Re Holliday* (A Bankrupt) (1981 Ch 405) where the children were 14, 9 and 6, there was a delay of five years. The petition in bankruptcy had been a tactical move by the husband to avoid a transfer of property in favour of his ex-wife. However, in the case of *Re Lowrie* (1981 3 AE 353) the sale at first instance was postponed for 30 months, there being children of three and a half years and one year old, but on appeal an immediate sale was ordered because it was held that the wife would have £10,000 from her share of the proceeds and even a lengthy delay would not change the situation so far as the children were concerned for they would still be very young.

The principle of marshalling will be of practical use to the spouse of a bankrupt. This means that particular secured debts may be applied only to the bankrupt's share of a property so that the spouse's share may be unaffected. For example, if an overdraft is secured on the matrimonial home by the bankrupt, having been obtained for his or her former business, marshalling would reduce the trustee in bankruptcy's share in the property by the amount of the overdraft. This would not, however, be possible if a new mortgage had been taken out merely to replace an older one, because it would be considered to be a debt incurred for the family's expenditure. It could not therefore be set only against the estate of the bankrupt but also against the share of the other spouse.

Chapter 9

Housing and property

Where the matrimonial home is owned, perhaps the most valuable single right a divorcing person has is to establish the proportion of it to which he or she is entitled and have it transferred (Section 24 Matrimonial Causes Act 1973); and, while the marriage is continuing, the right to occupy it under Section 2 of the Matrimonial Homes Act 1983 if the other spouse is the legal owner, that is to say if the deeds are in his or her name. Right of occupation can be registered at the Land Charges Registry if the property is not registered land, and at the Land Registry it is registered by entering a caution against dealings with it. If the home is rented the position is different; where it is rented from a local authority the possibility of a transfer of the tenancy is restricted.

Where a matrimonial home is rented the husband or wife considering divorce will need advice as to the kind of protection which may be available. There are very many different forms of occupation of land and references to them in this chapter, apart from what is said in the following paragraph, are limited to those relevant in the context of matrimonial breakdown.

Someone who is permitted to live on premises when not a tenant may be a licensee. This means that he or she has no security, as for example in the common situation of a couple living in the home of the parents of one of them. The permission can be withdrawn at any time. A licence is distinguishable from a tenancy, for which are required a landlord and a tenant, identifiable premises (even if the premises consist of a single room), a period of time, which may not be specified but which can be ended by the landlord or tenant, and exclusive possession. This last requirement means that the tenant has the use of the premises to the exclusion of others. It may be a matter of debate whether the occupation is a tenancy or a licence.

For instance, where a couple occupies a self-contained flat within the home of a parent in exchange for payment it is more likely to be a tenancy.

Local authorities and other providers of public housing, for example new town corporations and housing action trusts – and housing associations before 15 January 1989 – grant secure tenancies. The security they give is similar to tenancies in the private sector which are called assured tenancies. The landlord has to be one of the above bodies. A tenant is an individual occupying the property as his or her only or principal home. Exceptions include those occupying premises as employees and certain categories of homeless who may, however, be secured tenants if notified during the first year of the tenancy. A secured tenancy is lost if there is a change of landlord to one not included in the above categories or if the tenant ceases to occupy the property as his or her only or principal home. The tenancy may be ended by an outright or suspended possession order.

Under the domestic violence legislation it has been shown that the wife has the right to protection against her husband by a non-molestation order and sometimes an ouster order. The effect of these orders on private tenancies is not to deprive the husband of his tenancy, this being in the nature of a property right. In the short term a man evicted under an ouster order has little choice of accommodation. A men's hostel or rented bedsit is the only option if arrangements with family or friends cannot be made.

Since the Housing (Homeless Persons) Act 1977 local authorities have had a duty to help homeless people (now the statutory pro-vision is contained in the 1985 Housing Act). However, the gravity of the nationwide shortage of housing means that there is no long-term solution to the problem. The number of people accepted as homeless has increased in recent years (see the Law Commission publication *Domestic Violence and Occupation of the Family Home*, 1992) and the action of a local authority will depend upon whether someone is considered to be intentionally homeless or in priority need of housing. A woman can still be said to be homeless if she is living in a hostel (*Re London Borough of Ealing ex parte Sidhu* 1982) or if she is at risk of violence or the threat of violence from someone with whom she lives.

The effect of the Matrimonial Homes Act 1983 is to give both parties a right to occupy their home during the marriage, that is to say until decree absolute. Suspension of the right of one of them to occupy under Section 9(1) of the Act is, similarly, a short-term remedy. It seems unlikely that the removal of one party could be permitted by what is called a 'prohibited steps order' under Section 8(1) of the Children Act 1989. If there are divorce proceedings the court can, after decree nisi, order a transfer of the tenancy under Section 24 of the Matrimonial Causes Act but it will not take effect until decree absolute. It is vital that in the case of the wife of a violent husband an application for legal aid for ancillary relief is made as soon as a divorce petition is filed.

In the case of local authority housing the local authority landlord can transfer the tenancy, but the authority is unlikely to be willing to do so if there are rent arrears; and the husband cannot under the Matrimonial Homes Act be evicted permanently while the marriage subsists. The local authority has the right to be served with the ancillary relief application and if the court makes an order on decree nisi it should declare that the husband has no further right in the property.

Another legislative power which enables a transfer of tenancy to be ordered is conferred by Schedule 1 of the Matrimonial Homes Act 1983. This schedule also enables assured tenancies – the category which includes most private tenancies – to be transferred.

Problems can arise after decree nisi if one spouse has the possibility of a local authority flat. Although it is more convenient for the wife of a violent husband to have a transfer effected by the local authority, if the husband is in occupation after decree absolute there is a problem in enforcement because a warrant to enforce cannot be obtained in those circumstances. One wife who had a tenancy in her sole name throughout the marriage was able to obtain an injunction which excluded the husband from the property after decree absolute and before his application for ancillary relief was heard (*Lucas* v. *Lucas* 1992 2 FLR 53). This arose because the property was in her sole name, because the Matrimonial Homes Act applies to a spouse and an application under the Domestic Violence and Matrimonial Proceedings Act can be made when a couple are living in the same household as husband and wife. Where young children may be disturbed it may be possible to invoke the court's jurisdiction after decree absolute (*Quince* v. *Quince* (1983 4 FLR 394) and *Wild* v. *Wild* (1988 2 FLR 1983).

Where an order has been made post decree nisi and pre decree absolute it should be endorsed with a penal notice. This states that if the person to whom it is addressed does not obey it within the time limit contained in the order he or she will be liable to committal proceedings, that is a prison sentence. The order can then be enforced with a warrant for possession.

For most separated families the greatest fear is that marriage breakdown will be followed by homelessness. The duty of local authorities to provide accommodation is limited by the 1985 Housing Act. Their obligation to provide housing arises, as described above, when the authority is satisfied that the person seeking help is homeless and in priority need of accommodation. The test of priority need under Part 3 of the 1985 Act is satisfied if the person has dependent children, is homeless as a result of flood or fire, or if the person or anyone with him or her is vulnerable. Dependent children are those in full-time education or otherwise under the age of 16. The policy is explained in the *Code of Guidance* (DOE 1994) issued by the Secretary of State for the Environment. When in need of assistance from a local authority an applicant will need the *Code* in order to consider whether it has been applied by the local authority to which he or she has applied for housing. For instance the *Code* states that families should not be split, even for short periods.

Where an applicant is not considered to be in priority need the local authority has an obligation to provide advice and assistance. This may simply mean providing a list of housing associations and accommodation agencies. There may be a permanent housing obligation if the applicant is homeless and in priority need and the local authority is not satisfied that he or she became homeless intentionally. It may mean, however, that the obligation is related to the ability the authority has to refer the case to another authority.

The definition of homelessness and the question of intentional homelessness has given rise to many court decisions. A person is considered to be threatened if he or she is likely to become homeless within 28 days (Section 58(4) Housing Act 1985). However, homelessness arising from a possession order made as a result of non-payment of mortgage arrears is likely to be intentional homelessness. Temporary housing in a refuge was recognised as homelessness in the case referred to above (*Re London Borough of Ealing ex parte Sidhu* 1982).

Most tenancies in the private sector are assured tenancies, and since 15 January 1989 they have included housing association tenancies: they can be ended on certain statutory grounds under the 1988 Housing Act. A spouse who wishes a tenancy to be transferred needs to make an ancillary relief application to the court.

The interaction of criminal law and tenancies may also be of relevance. The Matrimonial Homes Act provides that without a court order the owner or tenant spouse cannot evict a non-owner or non-tenant spouse. And if a spouse is deserted, the Protection from Eviction Act enables him or her to remain subject to the remedies mentioned above.

For home-owning couples marriage breakdown entails decisions about selling the matrimonial home or retaining it on terms which will enable the departing spouse to receive a share of it then or later. The clean break discussed in Chapter 7 is possible when one spouse can afford to transfer to the other his or her share in the equity of the house. Clean breaks have been encouraged by the courts but seem less 'fashionable' now. When a wife is financially dependent it may be appropriate for her to agree to buy out a husband's share by increasing the mortgage. But many wives are low earners who will be unable to take on an additional mortgage without a guarantee of repayment from a relative who is prepared to pay if they cannot. Where the basis for a clean break is that low or no maintenance is paid for children and the wife later loses her job and is forced to obtain income support, mortgage interest may be paid by housing benefit; but the Child Support Agency will intervene on behalf of the children to obtain a child maintenance assessment against the father. The result may be the loss of housing benefit and a debt burden increased by mortgage interest.

Whichever party owns the property, the court has the power to vary property rights, but where a house is owned in the name of only one of them it is essential that the other protects himself or herself by registering a notice against the title under the Matrimonial Homes Act 1983 (Section 1). This notice against the registered title is notice to any prospective purchaser or lender of the occupation by the other. In order to register the notice the husband or wife has to find out the title number of the property. This is done by completing a Land Registry search form. The application to register a caution to obtain the protection is made on Land Registry form 63, citing the number of the property. Both forms are sold at law stationers' bookshops in major towns.

In the case of unregistered land the protection is acquired by application to the Land Charges Registry in Plymouth on a printed form for a Class F charge to be registered against the title. It can be cancelled on decree absolute so it is essential to pursue the financial application before that date. Such protection is not available if the property is owned by a company, even if the spouse is the majority shareholder, a company being a different legal entity.

Where the house is in joint names neither can sell without the agreement of the other, or a court order. The basis upon which property is jointly owned is that there exists a trust or binding obligation to sell. This can cause a problem where a couple have agreed to divorce two years after their physical separation and the one remaining in occupation is uncooperative about selling. It is possible to apply to the court for an order for sale under Section 30 of the Law of Property Act or Section 17 of the Married Women's Property Act 1882 provided the applicant is content to share the proceeds equally, because neither of these Acts gives the court the power to vary property rights. Even when such an order is made it is difficult for the absent spouse to ensure that conscientious attempts are made to sell the property by the one remaining in occupation. The absent spouse may ask the court to take this factor into account by giving him or her a larger slice of the property in the financial order; or he or she may consider that the basis of the separation agreement has been so undermined that an earlier divorce using adultery or unreasonable behaviour as evidence of breakdown would be justified.

Joint ownership may be in the form of what is known as a joint tenancy or a tenancy in common. Ownership by joint tenants entitles the surviving spouse to inherit the whole property. Such an outcome is often undesirable.

A tenancy in common gives each party a share, the amount of which depends upon their agreement. Either party can then leave his or her share to someone other than the spouse. A joint tenancy can be converted into a tenancy in common by the simple expedient of serving on the other party a notice stating that the joint tenancy has been severed and registering it with the Land Registry in the case of registered property (see Appendix 1 for form of notice). The Land Registry requires to be satisfied that the notice has been served on the other party. The effect of a tenancy in common is that one owner cannot give a receipt for the sale proceeds. If a tenancy in common exists, when one party dies the other will be forced to sell unless he or she inherits by the other's will, or the will provides for his or her right to occupy it during his or her lifetime.

Where the court makes an order for the sale or transfer of property and one spouse does not obey its terms by refusing to sign a contract for sale or to execute the transfer, an application can be made to the court for an officer of the court to execute the document. An order for costs of the application is likely to be made against the party who has disobeyed the court order.

Where an application is made in relation to a property it is essential under the Family Proceedings Rules 1991 (as amended) to serve the mortgagees with a copy of the notice of the application. This enables the mortgagees to indicate to the court whether they approve the proposals made by the petitioner or the respondent in advance of the court's decision. It would be disastrous for an order to be made transferring the property from one spouse to another subject to an existing mortgage if the mortgagees were not satisfied that the new owner of the entire property was able to discharge the burden of mortgage repayments.

The importance of establishing the size of a share in the family home cannot be too strongly emphasised. In a recent case (*McHardy & Sons* v. *Warren* 1994, *The Times* 8 April CA) the house was bought in the husband's name only but with the help of a £650 deposit, a wedding present from the wife's father. The Court of Appeal decided that the house was held for both husband and wife jointly and since the wife lived in it the creditors could not force the sale (see Chapter 8 on insolvency).

The mortgage may be collaterally secured by an endowment policy with an insurance company. The mortgage company may have suggested this form of security,which means that the borrower pays premiums on the insurance policy, which is taken out for the same amount as the mortgage. The borrower pays interest only on the mortgage instead of repaying capital as well, which would be the case in a repayment mortgage. During the period of the mortgage the insurance policy will increase in value until its maturity date when the capital of the mortgage will be repaid from it. If the policy is without profits it will produce sufficient to repay the mortgage. If it is with profits it will be expected to produce an additional figure, the amount of which depends upon vagaries of the market during the currency of the policy.

The policy may be in one or joint names and there may be more than one policy when the couple have borrowed additional monies during the course of their ownership in order to improve the property. The policies may have considerable value depending on the number of years for which they have been in existence, and the surrender value of such policies is included in the assets to be divided on divorce. Although they can be surrendered to provide immediate cash they may be of more value to the party who retains them as security for alternative borrowing for another property.

During the marriage the couple may have acquired a second home in England and Wales or abroad. Transfers of any property during the financial year in which a couple separate do not attract capital gains tax liability. After the year, the transfer of a property may have to be declared for capital gains tax purposes unless it falls within what is called Extra-Statutory Concession D6. This applies where the property is transferred by a person who had continued to occupy it and has not treated any other property as his or her principal residence. The calculation for capital gains tax is made on the basis set out on p. 139.

Chapter 10

Benefits for divorced and separated people

Gareth Morgan

SEPARATION

Separation, which for benefits purposes is a far more important situation than divorce, can often happen with little or no warning, throwing one or both parties into unexpected financial waters. This chapter attempts to guide the reader to the most important benefits which are likely to be relevant to recently separated people.

For the purpose of benefits, separation may occur when two people are still living together in the same house but no longer share their lives. If two people who were previously a couple, whether married or not, cease to maintain a joint household they become separate claimants for benefits.

BENEFITS

The benefits system in the UK is complex and administered by different central and local government agencies.

Department of Social Security: Through the Benefits Agency this is the central government department which administers and pays most benefits.
The Employment Service: This department administers the unemployment benefits system and operates the Job Centres network which provides employment and benefits advice.
Local authorities: The district councils and metropolitan authorities administer the housing benefits schemes. These consist of rent rebates and allowances for those paying rent for their homes and council tax benefit for council tax payers.

There are three main types of benefits.

Means tested or income-related benefits

These are normally the most important types of benefit and are designed to provide a safety net for those in greatest need. They are available to almost everybody who can show that they need them.

They include *income support* for people who are not in full-time work, *family credit* for those people who have children and who are in full-time work and *housing benefits* for people paying rent or council tax whether or not in full-time work. Full-time work for benefits purposes means 16 hours a week or more. There is also a benefit called *disability working allowance* for disabled people in full-time work but which there is not space here to examine in detail.

Contributory benefits

These are benefits which depend upon the claimant's record of national insurance contributions. These are the stamps which most people pay when in work, or which can be credited to them when they are sick or unemployed, or looking after children. The benefits for which they can qualify someone, depending on the number and type of contributions, include *unemployment benefit, sickness and maternity benefits* and *retirement pensions*.

Conditional and disability benefits

These are benefits which depend upon the claimant meeting some condition. For example *child benefit* is dependent upon having children, whom the applicant cares for and who are below a certain age and still at school. *Disability benefits* normally depend upon complex medical evidence and sometimes upon the cause of the disability, as do *industrial injuries benefits*.

Changes

Benefit rates normally increase in April each year but rule changes are frequent and the reader should always seek the current information from the relevant authority or from an advice agency or Citizens' Advice Bureau.

An example of change is the introduction of an earnings

disregard for childcare costs for those under 11 in registered care. This change occurred in October 1994 and had a considerable effect on the amount payable for several benefits.

All the amounts and figures quoted here are those for the 1996–97 benefits year.

MEANS TESTED BENEFITS

These important benefits are frequently the only benefits immediately available after the breakdown of a relationship and should be claimed where there is even a possibility of entitlement as soon as is possible. This is because they normally cannot be paid for any period before a claim form is submitted even when the claimant would have been entitled to receive them.

Income support

This is available for people who are not working or who work for less than 16 hours a week. If a couple is claiming, neither of them must work for 16 hours a week or more. Income support cannot be paid if there is more than £8,000 of capital and savings, excluding the value of the home and any personal possessions. Like all the means tested benefits, it depends upon a calculation of how much the claimant needs and how much income and capital they have.

How much is needed to live on is a figure called the applicable amount and is the total of several possible items.

Personal allowances

The first element is the personal allowances. This is determined by the number and ages of the people in the family. The amount for adults depends upon whether there is a single person or a couple (married or living together), and there is even an allowance for polygamous marriages. For example the personal allowance for a single claimant aged 25 or over is £47.90.

The amount for any children living in the family depends upon age. There are four age bands: under 11; 11 to 15; 16 and 17; 18 years old.

If the child is 16 or older, he or she must also be still at school or receiving equivalent non-advanced education such as at sixth-form college or an ONC course.

The 1996–97 benefit rates are found in Table 10.1 at the end of this chapter.

Premiums

These are amounts which recognise special needs of various sorts.

There are premiums for disability and severe disability where disability benefits are received for the adults or children or where someone is registered blind or meets other conditions.

There are age related premiums where people are aged over 60, 75 or 80.

There is a carers' premium for someone looking after a person who is getting attendance allowance or disability living allowance.

There is a lone parent premium where the claimant is a single parent.

The family premium is included where there are one or more children in the family.

Where a person qualifies for more than one of the disability, age or lone parent premiums, only the highest-value one is paid.

Housing

A new and more complicated method of dealing with income support for mortgages was introduced in October 1995. Most of the following rules do not apply to people who are aged over 60.

There are now different rules for those who were already paying for their home with a mortgage before 2 October 1995 and those who take out a mortgage for the first time after that date. However, mortgages taken out after 2 October 1995 will still be treated as if they had been taken out earlier for the purposes of the new rules, where the claimant;

has a child and has claimed income support because of the death of or the abandonment by a partner. This applies until the claimant becomes a member of a couple;

is not required to be available for employment because he or she is caring for a disabled person;

is in custody awaiting trial or sentence;

has been refused payment under a mortgage protection insurance policy because the claimant either has HIV or the insurance claim has been refused because of a pre-existing medical condition.

There is now a formula which is used to determine the amount of income support that will be paid towards the interest on a loan. If the actual amount of interest chargeable is less than 5 per cent, the actual interest rate will be met, otherwise a standard percentage interest rate is used, currently 7.74 per cent.

There is a limit of £100,000 maximum on which help will be given. There will be no income support for the first eight weeks of the claim in these circumstances.

Where a mortgage is taken out after 2 October 1995 there will be no help with housing costs from income support until the claimant has been receiving the benefit for a continuous period of 39 weeks.

The government has said that it believes home owners should take out insurance to cover them for what they say is normally a short period in receipt of benefit.

Resources

There are special rules which decide how much of a person's income is taken into account for income support.

Earnings

The earnings which are counted are the gross earnings less any tax or national insurance payable on them and less *half* of any occupational or private pension scheme contributions.

If there are any earnings from childminding, only one-third of them are counted.

Once the net earnings have been calculated an additional disregard is applied to the earnings, that is normally £5 of each person's earnings. There is a higher earnings disregard of £15 for a single parent or where there is a disability premium entitlement or where there are certain kinds of earnings such as reserve forces pay.

Other income

Most other income, such as child benefit and lone parent benefit is taken into account in full but there are some kinds of income, such as disability benefits, which are ignored in full and some, such as War Widows' Pensions, which are partially disregarded. There are special rules for income from boarders and sub-tenants.

Capital

If there are savings and capital under the limit of £8,000 but over £3,000 then a special notional income is assumed to exist. The actual value of any interest or income from capital is ignored and instead a tariff income is calculated where each £250 or part of over £3,000 is assumed to produce an income of £1 a week. For example a building society account with £4065.27 in it is assumed to produce a weekly income of £5. The £1,065.27 over the £3,000 starting point is four complete £250 units and one partial one, each of which produces £1 tariff income.

The amount payable

Income support is payable if the applicable amount (the needs figure) is more than the resources (the income figure). The amount payable is the difference between the sums.

Family credit

This is designed to help people who work for 16 hours a week or more and who have one or more children. It is payable for 6 months at a time after being claimed, regardless of any change of circumstance. This means that if it is the end of March when you qualify for family credit it may be better to wait until rates increase in early April before claiming. Similarly, if you know that your earnings will fall in the very near future you should consider delaying a claim.

Family credit sets a target figure which is made up of an allowance for adults, whether a couple or a single parent: this is £46.45 in the year 1996–97. There are allowances for children based on the same four age ranges as income support, although the amounts differ. The needs figure is increased by £10 where the claimant works for 30 hours a week or more.

The income rules are similar to income support but there are no disregards from the net earnings figure and child benefit is ignored as income.

The amount payable is worked out by comparing the income figure with a threshold amount of £75.20 in the year 1996–97. If the income figure is lower than that, the needs figure is payable in full; if the income is higher, the needs figure is reduced by 70p for each £1 of income by which the threshold figure is exceeded. At some point in this process the amount calculated will fall below 50p and family credit is not payable.

Housing benefits

These benefits provide help to people who pay rent and/or council tax. This includes boarders and sub-tenants as well as people renting their home from a private landlord, housing association or council. Rent rebates apply to people renting from councils and are awarded as a discount on the rent payable. Rent allowances apply to all others and are normally paid to the tenant, although they can be paid to the landlord in some circumstances. The calculations are identical for the two benefits except that the council can decide that the rent payable for rent allowances is too high and limit the amount on which benefit is payable.

Council tax benefit can be applied for by anyone who pays council tax.

There are no restrictions on the hours of work for any housing benefits but there is a limit of £16,000 for capital and savings above which you cannot receive the benefits.

The applicable amounts calculation is the same as that for income support except that the one parent premium is higher. There are also more generous disregards of earnings for lone parents.

Eligible rent

The rent on which housing benefit is calculated may not be the amount which is actually being paid.

From the beginning of January 1996 the government has introduced changes to decide how much rent housing benefit can help with.

'A local reference rent' is set by the rent officer and is the average of the highest and lowest reasonable rents for that kind of property in that area. Housing benefit will be paid up to the level of that rent. If the actual rent payable is more than that, housing benefit will pay only half of the difference. The local authority has some discretion to pay more if exceptional hardship would be caused, but in practice it may be difficult to persuade them to do this. People who already receiving housing benefit in January 1996 will be exempted from this calculation until their circumstances change.

At the same time the government introduced a scheme to allow tenants to receive 'pre-tenancy determinations'. This means that somebody considering taking on a tenancy will, with the consent of the landlord, be able to ask the local authority to provide them with a figure within very few days of the eligible rent on which housing benefit will be based. This figure will not be the amount of housing benefit actually payable but will be the maximum rent figure that housing benefit could meet. The 'local reference rent' scheme does not apply to local authority or housing association properties.

Some things covered by the rent paid may not be eligible for help. These include ineligible service charges for items such as food, heating, nursing help and cleaning.

A deduction may also be made for anybody other than the adults and qualifying children who live in the house. If the claimant is a boarder there will be a deduction for the contribution made towards the water and sewerage charges of the building.

In a shared ownership scheme, where a person pays rent and also has a mortgage on part of the house, income support may help with the mortgage interest payments and housing benefit is available for the rental part of the payments.

Eligible council tax

Most people will normally be entitled to apply for help towards the council tax they pay but there may be deductions for anybody other than the adults and qualifying children who live in the house. There is a very complex calculation called 'second adult rebate' which may need to be carried out if there are other adults in the house. The council should do this automatically but the Citizens' Advice Bureau will be able to explain whether it applies.

Calculation

The amount payable is worked out by comparing the income figure with the amount calculated for needs. If the income figure is lower than that for needs then the eligible rent and council tax are payable in full, although the local authority has the power to limit the payment if they believe that the rent is too high. If the income is higher than the needs, then the rent rebate is reduced by 65p for each £1 of income by which the threshold figure is exceeded, and the council tax benefit by 20p for each £1. At some point in this process the amount calculated will fall below 50p and housing benefit will not be payable.

Child support, maintenance income and payments

Child support payments received are taken into account for all means tested benefits. They are counted in full for income support but there is a disregard of £15 a week for family credit, disability working allowance, housing benefit and council tax benefit.

Other maintenance payments received normally count in full for income support unless they fall into certain categories, which include payments in kind; school fees; money from the disposal of property after separation or divorce.

There are special rules which apply to lump sums but advice should be sought as capital is sometimes treated as income and the calculation is complex.

There is no longer any disregard of maintenance payments made by a claimant.

Child benefit

Child benefit is payable to the person with whom a child 'lives' or, sometimes, to a person who contributes to the maintenance of the child at, at least, the rate of child benefit for that child and who is considered to be the highest-priority person.
The priorities are:

the person with whom the child lives;
the wife, where husband and wife reside together and are not divorced or judicially separated;
a parent;
the mother, where both parents live together but are not married.

It is payable at the rate of £10.80 for the eldest child and £8.80 for each other child. One parent benefit of £6.30 is payable to those single people who are receiving child benefit.

New relationships

The effect of a new relationship upon benefits entitlement can be dramatic. Once a decision has been made that a couple are living together they become treated as a family and their financial situations are lumped together. If one of them is working for more than 16 hours a week all entitlement to income support is lost. Conversely, if there is a child, a decision that a couple are living together as husband and wife will allow family credit to be claimed.

If the parties disagree that they are living together then an appeal against the decision can be made, as described on pp. 93–4.

The mortgage

Help with mortgage payments is only available to people who receive income support. This means that all help with mortgage interest payments stops when somebody works for an average of 16 weeks or more. This is not the case with housing benefit, which is available to those paying rent, where the benefit tapers away gradually with increased income regardless of hours of work.

The effect of this is such that people with mortgages should consider the figures carefully before taking up work, especially low-paid work, as it is comparatively easy to be worse off in employment, particularly if there are no children and family credit cannot be claimed.

Pensions and the contribution record

Many benefits depend upon the amount and period of time for which national insurance contributions have been paid. The unemployment and sickness benefits schemes look at the two previous years of contributions but the retirement pensions scheme looks at a much longer period of time and this needs to be examined carefully by separated and divorced people. This is particularly important for wives who may not have worked for many years and who had been relying upon their husbands' contribution record.

There are rules which help people who are divorced and who do not qualify on their own contributions. If the person does not remarry before they reach pensionable age, or the decree absolute is granted after pensionable age, then the ex-spouse's contributions may be counted towards their contribution record. The rules about this are complex and advice should be sought, as there may be a choice between two methods of calculating contributions.

The effect of these rules may mean that there are advantages in not divorcing after separation if the former spouse is still working and paying contributions.

Social fund

The social fund makes one-off payments to people in need. There are two types of payment: grants which are available automatically if certain conditions are met, and discretionary grants or loans.

Mandatory grants

The automatic grants where income support, family credit or disability working allowance are being paid include a maternity grant. There must be capital of below £500 to receive the full grant of £100 and the claim must be made between 11 weeks before the expected date of confinement and three months after the birth. The grant can be claimed for stillborn children provided the pregnancy lasted 24 weeks and the grant can be made for adopting a child provided the claim is made within three months of the adoption. If family credit is claimed because of the birth of the child the grant should be claimed within the times above even if the family credit claim has not been decided.

The other automatic grants are for funeral expenses and for payments when there has been cold weather and there are young children or old or disabled people in the household.

Discretionary grants and loans

These are limited by the budget available to each office and there is no automatic entitlement to them. Most of the payments are loans which are normally repaid by deduction from benefit. There are certain guidelines which the officers should follow when deciding whether or not to make payments, but even where an application falls within these guidelines there is no guarantee of success. The £500 capital limit rule applies to these payments.

Community care grants can be made to people who receive income support for a number of reasons. These include people who are moving out of institutional or residential care, to help people not to enter such care, to ease exceptional pressure on families and for some travelling expenses.

The guidance suggests that grants could be given to help families move after the breakdown of relationships, especially if there has been violence; for children's clothing where there has been excessive wear and tear; for the costs of installing pre-payment meters where there are young children; and for minor repairs to the house where there are children. There is no comprehensive list of inclusions or exclusions and the best advice is to claim if there is a need.

Travelling expenses can be paid to visit people who are ill, to attend relatives' funerals, to ease domestic crises and to visit a child living with the other parent pending a court decision on who is to have responsibility for the child. These can include overnight expenses where the distances justify it.

Loans, which are interest free, are available to help with budgeting and crises.

Budgeting loans are available to those who have been getting income support for at least six months and are for amounts between £30 and £1,000. The types of item for which loans are available are divided into high, medium and low priorities. Examples of high-priority items are bedclothes and essential items of furniture, medium-priority includes clothing and inessential items of furniture while low-priority includes leisure items and rent in advance. The officer must decide that the applicant can afford to repay the loan.

Crises loans are available to people who do not get income support but who have suffered an emergency or disaster. It must be the only way of preventing damage or a serious risk to health or safety. The guidance gives fire and flood as examples of disaster.

Appeals

Where there is a disagreement over a decision about a benefit it is possible to ask for a review of the decision, and if that is unsatisfactory a formal appeal can be made. Legal aid is not available for tribunal representation but many advice agencies will provide representatives. An experienced representative will be helpful, as the appeal will probably require a good understanding of the law.

For income support, family credit and disability working allowance these appeals are heard by the Independent Tribunal

Service which provides a nationwide and efficient service, although the process can take a considerable time to complete. If there is disagreement with the appeal tribunal decision on a point of law, then the matter can go further, to a commissioner of social security and, if appropriate, as far as the House of Lords.

For housing benefit, an appeal is heard by a panel of local councillors who make up a housing benefit review board. Many of these are considered by experts to operate in an unsatisfactory manner but the only method of appeal from them is by asking for a judicial review, which is a difficult, complex and potentially expensive process.

Social Fund appeals on mandatory grant decisions go to the same tribunal as income support. Discretionary grants and loans have no right of appeal but a review can be asked for and if that is not satisfactory a Social Fund Inspector can be asked to carry out a further review.

Other entitlements

Once income support or family credit is being paid there are a number of other benefits which follow automatically, such as free prescriptions, optical and dental treatment and travel costs to hospital. Free school meals are received if income support is being paid.

There is also a means test for health benefits where people are not in receipt of income support or family credit; this is slightly more generous but almost as complex as the income support calculation. It is also much underused. It is worth enquiring or contacting an advice agency to check on entitlement on low-income grounds.

Free milk and vitamins are available to children under 5 where the family are on income support, and disabled children who cannot attend school receive free milk until the age of 16. People who get family credit and who have children under a year old can buy dried milk at a specially reduced price from child and maternity clinics.

ADVICE AND ASSISTANCE

Benefits is a complex area. Special rules and conditions abound and these are outside the scope of this chapter. It is strongly advised that advice is taken about individual circumstances. Citizens' Advice Bureaux, law centres and other advice agencies have a wealth of knowledge and experience of the benefits system and are usually much better at giving advice in this area than solicitors. The DSS provide many leaflets and operate a nationwide telephone enquiry line.

Table 10.1 Means tested benefit rates, April 1996–97

Income Support
Personal allowances

under 18 (usual rate)	£28.85
under 18 (in certain circumstances)	£37.90
aged 18–24	£37.90
aged 25 or over	£47.90
Single Parent	
under 18 (usual rate)	£28.85
under 18 (in certain circumstances)	£37.90
aged 18 or over	£47.90
Couple	
both under 18	£57.20
one/both over 18	£75.20
Dependent children	
under 11	£16.45
aged 11–15	£24.10
aged 16–17	£28.85
aged 18	£37.90

Premiums

	Single	Couple
Family		£10.55
Lone parent		£5.20
Pensioner	£19.15	£28.90
Enhanced pensioner	£21.30	£31.90
Higher pension	£25.90	£37.05
Disability	£20.40	£29.15
Severe disability	£36.40	£36.40 (if one qualifies) £72.80 (if both qualify)
Disabled child	£20.40	
Carer	£13.00	

Housing benefit
Personal allowances and premiums as for income support,

except single person aged 16–24	£37.90

continued.,

single parent under 18	£37.90
lone parent premium	£11.50

Council tax benefit
Personal allowances and premiums as for
income support,
except lone parent premium	£11.50

Family Credit
Adult credit	£46.45
Child credit	
under 11	£11.75
aged 11–15	£19.45
aged 16–17	£24.15
aged 18	£33.80
Applicable amount (i.e. threshold level)	£75.20

Disability Working Allowance
Adult credit	
single	£48.25
couple/loan parent	£75.60
Child credit	
under 11	£11.75
aged 11–15	£19.45
aged 16–17	£24.15
aged 18	£33.80
Applicable amount (i.e. threshold level)	
single	£56.40
couple/lone parent	£75.20
disabled child's allowance	£20.40

Chapter 11

Maintenance of children

In 1993 a new administrative system was introduced by the Child Support Act of 1991 for assessing maintenance in all new cases of the children of separated families. The Child Support Agency provides an administrative system which has a jurisdiction parallel to that of the court system, which continues to deal with child support in areas not covered by the Act. It also continues to deal with capital for children and with spousal claims for maintenance and capital.

The new system was set up to provide for the assessment, collection and enforcement of maintenance for children under the age of 19 who are not in advanced education, that is to say university education, who have not been married, and who do not live, and neither of whose parents live, habitually abroad. It does not include stepchildren and in a society of serial marriages this means that different children of the same family are often treated differently with respect to maintenance, a result wholly at odds with the objective of the Children Act 1989, which was to treat similarly children of the same family.

Another major difference between the Child Support Act and the Children Act is that the former gives paramountcy to the children whereas in the Child Support Act their welfare is merely a factor to which a child support officer may have regard.

The objectives of the new system were set out in the Government White Paper *Children Come First* (Command Number 1263 1990). It sought to create a consistent pattern of maintenance for children throughout the country based on a formula system as distinct from the discretion-based system of the courts. It was intended that there should be a reduction in social security benefit expenditure from the improved arrangement and it was expected that parents on benefit would also enjoy an improvement in their position.

State involvement in supporting many separated families through the benefits system is very expensive. The 'liable relatives' provisions of the social security legislation prior to the implementation of the child support legislation enabled the Department of Social Security to pursue non-paying absent parents for maintenance, but the returns were unsatisfactory. Few could quarrel with the proposition that the state should recover what was paid out provided that the absent parents could meet their responsibilities appropriately.

The operation of the new system has given rise to great disquiet, not least on the part of absent parents whose high incomes initially led to much higher child maintenance assessments than the amounts they would have been ordered to pay in the courts system. The parents with care, as those who have the children living with them most of the time are called, have been relatively silent on the issue, but the government claims that many of them have been able, as a result of assessments in excess of income support, to float off income support, into work that earns a realistic income. However, more than a fivefold increase in unpaid child maintenance from £95 million to £525 million between March 1994 and March 1995 was reported in June 1995 and the Permanent Secretary at the Department of Social Security announced for 1996 the target of reducing the measure of errors in assessment to one in four. It was conceded by the Permanent Secretary that the Treasury rather than the child was the 'primary financial beneficiary of the new system'.

Changes made by regulations in February 1994 removed some of the opposition to the Act by reducing the additional element in higher-income cases where there were fewer than three children of the family. At the same time a standard figure in the calculation of what is called 'protected income' (the level against which no parent shall pay more) was increased from £8 to £30 per week to ensure that a parent is left with greater income than would be the case if he or she were on benefit. These changes combined to relieve both better-off absent parents and those in very straitened circumstances.

At issue, however, is the question of the right of the state to adjudicate in disputes between two individuals in the place of the court if no question of benefits is involved. Article 6(2) of The European Convention on Human Rights provides for 'a fair public hearing' in the determination of everyone's civil rights and obligations. It is not possible for a litigant in England and Wales who is aggrieved by a decision here to make an application to the European Court without first exhausting the possible remedies here. This may mean that someone aggrieved by a decision of the Child Support Agency will have to go through the administrative system – that is to say make an appeal to the Child Support Appeal Tribunal and then to the Child Support Commissioner and, if a point of law is concerned, to the Court of Appeal – before contemplating an application to the European Court. Alternatively, it may be possible to challenge the administrative decisions of the Agency or the Tribunal or the Commissioner by making an application in the High Court for judicial review of the decision. Some challenges by this system have resulted in a settlement of the disputed issue but there are very few reported decisions.

It is obviously sensible to avoid invoking the jurisdiction of the Agency by reaching an agreement on the amount of child maintenance as well as other matters. The new system complicates negotiations for agreement for two reasons. First the agreement made on all issues may be recorded in a separation agreement but the Child Support Act (Section 9) provides that a written agreement should not prevent any parent making an application to the Child Support Agency for an assessment.

Secondly, where a couple can afford a clean break on capital, and perhaps income, sometimes on the basis that the wife gets more or all of the equity in the house, such a break is of benefit to the whole family because the husband can start afresh and the wife, when the children are adults, may be able to sell the property and have some money left to invest or add to her pension contributions if she has not made the maximum possible contribution to her scheme.

If, however, she loses her job and becomes dependent on income support in circumstances where it has been agreed that the husband shall not pay her maintenance or very little, the Agency has the power to make an assessment in respect of the children. Maintenance may be being paid to the children but if it is less than the formula would produce it will be superseded.

Settlement negotiations are therefore considerably complicated by the new system. Most good solicitors should have acquired computer systems to enable them to calculate the assessment the formula imposed by the Act would produce. Such calculations are necessary if the court is to make a determination on the other maintenance and capital claims before an assessment is made. A redistribution of capital and income for the family will inevitably result in a change of circumstances, justifying a new assessment.

Subject to these caveats it is still better to try and reach an agreement which will result in a consent order sealed by the court. However, absent parents (as they are called by the legislation) who retain a share of their former matrimonial home as a result of the negotiations will need to be aware of the possibility of a capital gains tax liability arising when the property is sold, because the order is likely to provide for sale when the eldest child has left school or completed full-time education.

In cases which were decided before 5 April 1993 or which were already in the court system the orders made in relation to the maintenance of children will continue to have effect and applications to vary those orders can be made by the court until they are taken over by the Agency.

The Agency takeover of all cases, which was to have taken place between April 1996 and April 1997, has been deferred, as has the take-on of income support cases where court orders were made before 1993. The reason for the deferment is the volume of work with which the Agency has been overwhelmed. Delays are inevitable and mistakes are the rule rather than the exception.

Following the report of the House of Commons Select Committee on Social Security in October 1994, which recommended certain changes to the formula, the government produced the White Paper *Improving Child Support* (HMSO 1995) which anticipated further changes to the legislation. These have now been made. Regulations which took effect in April 1995 provided that absent parents should be left with at least 70 per cent of their net income, income being calculated according to the child support formula. It was also stated that an absent parent will not pay more than 33 per cent in a combination of current liability and start-up arrears. The whole of an absent parent's housing costs will be allowed as part of his or her exempt income, instead of a proportion, as was formerly the case where he or she had formed a new relationship and had a second family. Interest payments on unpaid maintenance assessments were abolished but will be replaced in 1997 with a system of penalties for late payments. Fees are not payable for two years from April 1995. Property and capital settlements – provided that they meet certain conditions, of which the principal one is that they should not have been made in settlement of an adult's claims for maintenance – can be taken into account in allowing a parent to pay less. A further change is an allowance of 10p per mile for travel to work costs in excess of 150 miles per week. In a case where a parent travels 200 miles per week his or her assessable income will be reduced by £5 per week. In most cases where the assessment is calculated on the basis of what is called the 'basic element' the assessment is made from half of the assessable income so that the amount of travel will result in a reduction in the assessment of £2.50 per week. There has also been a softening of the effects of the legislation in allowing for an assessment not to start for eight weeks following the date when an enquiry form was sent out to an absent parent: previously the liability arose from the date when the form was dispatched.

A new Act, the Child Support Act 1995 has been passed to provide a system of departure from the standard formula which is described below. This enables either parent to apply to a child support officer on the grounds that because he or she faces additional expenses not covered by the formula they would suffer hardship as a result of the formula being applied. The kinds of additional expenses likely to qualify are exceptionally high travel costs to work, high travel costs to maintain contact with the children, expenses of disability, certain debts of the former relationship, some pre-1993 debts and in some cases the costs of caring for stepchildren. Capital and property settlements made before 1993 will be a ground for applying for departure from the formula when a test of fairness to both parents would be used. At the time of writing it is expected that the draft regulations, which were published in the spring of 1996, and define the departure provisions will be very restrictively applied.

The appeals system established by the legislation has not worked very satisfactorily. An appeal is made initially after a child support officer has checked the decision of the officer who made the assessment by a child support appeal tribunal consisting of a legally qualified chairman or chairwoman and two lay members. Under the first Act they were not able to replace wrong assessments with correctly calculated ones; they will be able to do so under the new Act in departure cases. Further appeals are to a child support commissioner, very few of whose decisions have been published. An appeal can be made on a point of law from a commissioner to the Court of Appeal. Where there has been a substantial irregularity the decision of the Agency can be challenged by an application for leave to have the decision judicially reviewed by a divisional court of the Queen's Bench. Subject to eligibility, legal aid can be obtained for the application for leave and for the application itself if leave is given. It is usually expected that if there is a point on which an appeal could have been made the appeal procedure should first be exhausted.

The main problem where there has been more than one marriage breakdown is how the children of the family will be treated. If a wife has two children by her first marriage, and she obtained a court order for their maintenance before April 1993, or subsequently by agreement with her ex-husband, her case will not be taken on by the Agency. If she did not have an order she will be obliged to seek an assessment from the Agency if she has insufficient maintenance, and if she is in receipt of state benefits the Agency will itself apply for an assessment. When she petitions for divorce from her second husband she will be able to make a claim for maintenance for the same children of her first marriage against her second husband on the basis that her second husband contributed to the support of his stepchildren. Ironically, she cannot claim in the petition for maintenance for the natural children of her second husband but will have to apply to the Agency unless maintenance is agreed.

If the second husband had children by a first marriage he will probably be paying maintenance under a court order if he was divorced from his first wife before the new system came into effect. The amount he pays under the order is allowed for in the protected income calculation which limits the amount of income he pays following the assessment. If, however, the first and second marriage broke down after April 1993 there would be two sets of assessments under the formula, and the existence of the natural children of the first marriage would be acknowledged in the application of the formula to the maintenance application for the children of the second marriage.

Where an assessment does not produce sufficient maintenance for children in the view of the mother, an application can be made to the court for what is described as a 'top-up'. This is also the case where the expenses of a disabled child are involved and an order in relation to the costs resulting from disablement needs to be obtained from the court. Likewise an application for school fees has to be made to the court after the assessment has been made by the Agency.

A particular difficulty for most parents is the absence of legal aid and the unequal position of a parent who has no means and cannot obtain advice on the formula applying to his or her case. The Agency is bound by Civil Service rules of confidentiality and cannot disclose information about the absent parent's means other than what the assessable income is calculated to be (see p. 000) but it has access to information on the court file and government records including DSS records, the NHS computer and the Inland Revenue.

A petitioner who is on benefit has no choice about co-operating with the Agency in obtaining an assessment unless he or she succeeds in persuading the child support officer that harm or distress will be caused to him or her or any of the children living with him or her as a result of an assessment being made. Withholding information from a child support officer is punishable by reduction of 20 per cent of the income support personal allowance component (£47.90 per week) for six months and 10 per cent for a year. That means, at present rates, a reduction for six months of £9.30 per week and for a further year of £4.79 week.

The problem for a payer of a child support assessment is that the assessment applies eight weeks from the date that a maintenance enquiry form is sent to him. If no response is received a 14-day notice can be issued of the intention to impose an interim maintenance assessment. This will be at one and a half times the maintenance requirement. An interim maintenance assessment may be considerably higher than the assessment that would be imposed if the information about the payer's means had been available, but there is no regulation providing for repayment by the Agency of higher amounts although there is provision for the Agency to recover more maintenance if the interim maintenance assessment is not as high as the subsequent assessment. Some ameliorative changes are anticipated in 1996 to the administration of interim assessments.

A concern in the early days of the Agency was that voluntary payments of maintenance would be ignored when assessments were made. This is not supposed to be the case although many assessments have given rise to disputes that sums thus paid have been ignored.

The cause of most of the anger resulting from the operation of the Agency is that the assessments are based on a rigid formula. Amending regulations which came into force in February 1994 reduced the maintenance requirement where the children of the family were over 11 and further reduced it when they were over 13. By also reducing what is called the amount of the additional element paid by better-off fathers the changes disappointed the expectations which many parents with care, as the Act calls them, had of the system. The formula is constructed to calculate how much an absent parent should pay each week.

The Act, like the law on child maintenance applied by the courts, is based on the principle that both parties are responsible for maintaining their children. The formula divides the responsibility between them by ascertaining how much the absent parent should pay. Account is taken of both parents' assessable incomes where both parents have an assessable income. If an absent parent is out of work he or she will still be expected to contribute a minimum sum of £4.65 per week. The maintenance requirement is not a fixed amount for each child of the family because it is based on income support allowances, which are periodically reviewed. It consists of a number of components and the requirement for all the children of the family will depend on the number of children of the family and their ages. Their requirement consists of the aggregate of the amount for each qualifying child minus child benefit (but not the single parent addition). It includes the amount for the income support personal allowance for a child, the amount of the income support family premium plus, where one child is under 16, the amount of the adult income support personal allowance plus, where the parent with care has no partner, a lone parent premium. Where there are two children aged between 11 and 15 the maintenance requirement in 1995 was £78.28, calculated as follows:

Child allowance	
(2 children between 11 and 15) @ £23.40 each	£46.80
Adult allowance of carer	
(75 per cent of £46.50 because one child is 11)	34.88
Lone parent premium	5.20
Family premium	10.25
	£97.13
Less child benefit	18.85
	£78.28

Before the February changes the maintenance requirement for the two children (based on the April 1994 uprating) would have been £88.40.

The assessable income in each case is the net income of each parent less tax, national insurance and half his or her pension contributions. A deduction is then made in respect of exempt income. Exempt income consists of housing costs, the adult personal allowance and any applicable premiums and child allowances. Only half of an absent parent's assessable income is applied to meet his or her responsibility for maintaining the children for whom an assessment is made.

EXAMPLE

After deduction of tax, national insurance and half pension contributions James earns £200 net per week and has housing costs of £50 per week. His assessable income per week on 1995 rates will therefore be as follows:

Net income		£200.00
Less:		
housing costs	£50.00	
adult personal allowance	46.50	96.50
Assessable income		£103.50

Alison, James's wife, has a net weekly income after tax and national insurance and half her pension contributions of £221.30. Her housing costs are £80 in respect of her mortgage. Alison's assessable income will be:

Net income		221.30
Less:		
housing costs	80.00	
adult personal allowance	46.50	
family premium	5.20	
lone parent premium	10.25	
child allowances	46.80	188.75
Assessable income		£32.55

Because Alison's protected income will be £221.96 she has no assessable income.

It would be immaterial for the purpose of an assessment that James pays Alison's housing costs of £80 per week, because the only housing costs which are part of exempt income are those paid for the roof over one's own head. As a contribution towards his children's maintenance the Agency may give recognition of it. If the two children are under 11 their maintenance requirement would have been as follows in 1995:

Child allowances	
(two children under 11) 2 × 15.95	31.90
Family premium	10.25
Lone parent premium	5.20
Adult personal allowance	46.50
	93.85
Less child benefit	18.85
Maintenance requirement	75.00

But if both children are over 11 the adult allowance element which is intended to reflect their need for care is reduced by 50 per cent, and if both children are over 13 by 75 per cent, so that the maintenance requirement in the first case is reduced by £23.25 and in the second case by £34.88 per week.

The result in the assessment payable by James in the different cases would be as follows. Where both children are under 11 the maintenance requirement will be £75.00, and where both are over 11 and under 15 the maintenance requirement will be £66.65. The responsibility for meeting this is to be met from half the parents' assessable income. This will be £51.75 (£103.50 divided by 2). £51.75 is all that James can pay. He will be unable to meet £80 per week housing costs as well.

In cases of better-off families an additional element will apply. Thus if after the maintenance requirement is met from less than half the assessable income, an additional element of 15 per cent for one child and 20 per cent for two children is added. So if half James's assessable income were £200 per week after the maintenance requirement of £66.65 had been met there would be £133.35 left. Twenty per cent of this figure, £26.67, will be added to the assessment. If the regulations had not been amended the amount of the additional element at 25 per cent would have been £33.33.

Before an assessment is imposed a protected income test is made in respect of the payer's income in order to ensure that he appears to be left with a basic means of support. This test, while including a standard margin of £30 which is £22 higher than before February 1994, does not take into account or recognise the existence of other commitments.

Since the only housing costs which count are those for the roof over the parent's head there is some incentive for them to increase those housing costs in order to reduce the assessment which may be made, subject however to some restrictions imposed by the regulations.

There is no monitoring of assessments, so it is not known whether, as a result of meeting assessments made by the Agency, there are more possession actions by mortgagees in cases where families cannot continue to make their mortgage repayments. The practical effect of the Act for parents negotiating agreements for maintenance is first to calculate maintenance for the children based on the formula – in case one of them subsequently applies for an assessment – and only after that to calculate the amount of income support which should be available to the wife and children not affected by the legislation and capital questions. This is the reverse of the discretion-based system employed by the courts in which first the wife's needs were considered and then the needs of the children, based on their per capita needs. Perhaps the one positive aspect of the legislation has been that the real cost of caring for children has been given prominence but this is of little comfort to poor families, especially those on benefit who may not have benefited from the assessments made against the fathers of their children.

Claims for capital for children, even those under the Child Support legislation, can of course continue to be made to the court (Children Act 1989 Schedule 1). Maintenance for children at university will also be dealt with by the court. A little-noticed result of the separation of parents whose children are at university is that where a mother's means may entitle a child to a full grant the means of the father contributing then or subsequently to the support of the child is ignored. If the family had lived together the child might not have qualified at all for the grant. It is not known how many families benefit in this way but of course if maintenance is awarded to the wife on the reassessment of the entitlement to grant in the following year an adjustment will be made.

Chapter 12

Pensions and insurance

The pension which most people expect to receive is the state retirement pension for women from the age of 60 and for men from the age of 65, but women in employment after 2010 will not be so entitled until the age of 65. The state retirement pension has two parts. One is a flat rate, the full amount of which depends on the contributions to the national insurance scheme made by the pensioner while working or made on behalf of a woman by her husband. On divorce it is sensible to enquire of the Department of Social Security as to the level of additional national insurance contributions it may be necessary for a woman to make in order to maintain the maximum retirement pension.

In 1978 the government introduced the State Earnings Related Pension Scheme (SERPS) which is the second part of the state pension. This is intended to produce one-fifth of average earnings on retirement, but those working could contract out of the scheme in order to make their own arrangements by membership of a suitable pension scheme.

Many firms have occupational pension schemes which provide for the widow or widower of their members. The value of the loss of future pension benefit is one of the factors the court is obliged to take into consideration when making financial orders following divorce (Section 25 Matrimonial Causes Act 1973; see Chapter 7).

If an employee changes employment the pension rights from his or her previous earnings may remain in the former company's fund or may be transferred to the scheme of his or her new employers. The proportion of gross earnings which can be contributed to a pension depend on age: below the age of 50, 17.5 per cent of earnings can be contributed, tax relief being given at the top rate of tax so that there is considerable tax saving for those who are paying tax at 40 per cent. The proportion of earnings which can be made increases after the age of 50, so that by 60, 40 per cent can be contributed. A future pensioner paying income tax at 40 per cent making a contribution of £10,000 in one year, will if aged under 50, be relieved of tax on £1,750 of the sum because £1,750 of the earnings will be disregarded for income tax. The same contribution at the age of 60 will result in £4,000 of the sum being ignored for tax purposes.

The self-employed can make contributions to a variety of schemes by single premium pension policies or regular monthly payments towards such schemes. They often begin contributing relatively late in their working lives. The contributions made can reflect the earnings made during the last six financial years but, provided the funds are available, very large contributions can be made from time to time. Such a self-employment arrangement may or may not provide for a widow. Many such arrangements are made, usually by the decision of the future pensioner a short time before retirement. Those who are self-employed often take out insurance policies for dependent children which will not form part of their estate for inheritance tax purposes. Such arrangements will obviously be considered by the court when making decisions on ancillary relief applications.

In the past, divorced couples paid scant attention to the value of future pensions on a divorce. There are two categories now where loss of pension benefit is unlikely to be an issue because there is unlikely to be any loss: where there has been a short marriage and the husband's retirement is far off (*Hedges* v. *Hedges* 1991 1 FLR 196), or where the parties are young and the wife can pursue her own opportunities for career and pension.

A pension may be worth more than the matrimonial home but it is not an asset which can be assigned.

In 1985 the Lord Chancellor's Department recommended changes in the law to enable a wife to apply, on her former husband's death, for pension provision. This would mean continuing uncertainty for both following divorce. Recent suggestions have been made by the Institute of Fiscal Studies and the Labour Party for an equal division of pensions on divorce, but such a division would clearly not be fair in a case where the marriage had lasted for a small proportion of the working lifetime during which pension contributions were made.

The law does not permit pension-splitting at present. Germany has a pension-splitting system which is operated by the court, unless the parties have made their own agreement, which they often do if they have similar pension rights. Transfers of pension rights are effected by the German court when the necessary information has been obtained about each party's present and future pension rights. This is relatively simple if the parties are employed by the state. If the husband has a private pension scheme that cannot be split at the time of the divorce the wife has to pursue her former husband when he reaches retirement age. There are alternatives to full pension-splitting which involve the husband contributing to the wife's pension scheme and the right of a former wife to seek a pension if her husband dies before retirement, provided she would still, but for the divorce, have received a widow's pension.

The law in Scotland has been different from that in England and Wales since the Family Law (Scotland) Act of 1985 explicitly provided for pension and life insurance benefits to be included in matrimonial property; and the courts there have the power to order present or future payments in respect of pensions. There is no power for the husband to make payments into a personal pension scheme for the wife, a change which would give both parties tax advantages.

The Scottish experience since 1985 indicates that pensions are more likely to be used as bargaining counters and less likely to be valued. In 1991 the Law Society in England and Wales recommended legislation to provide powers for the courts to make pension adjustment orders at the time when it decides other financial questions following divorce as well as the power to allow payments by husbands into pension schemes for their wives. It also asked for guidance to be provided as to when a pension should be valued.

In 1993 the Pensions Management Institute (PMI) in agreement with the Law Society reported on pensions on divorce. The PMI report recommended that the court should be given certain limited powers. It proposed that the value of a pension should be measured by its cash equivalent, that is the basis of transfer values payable from one pension scheme to another. It looked at four ways of reallocating pension values: the adjustment of a couple's assets by giving the wife a bigger share of non-pension assets; by earmarking a proportion of pension rights for a former spouse payable when the pension became payable; by splitting the pension so that part of it was available for a former wife as a separate member of the scheme; and by releasing a proportion of the pension for the former wife to be transferred to another arrangement. This recommendation was made on the basis that the law could be changed to give the court power to require pension trustees to reduce the member's rights by a specified sum and make it available to the divorced spouse for a personal pension or to a scheme of which the divorced spouse was a member. It further recommended that if the divorce took place after the pension was in payment the court should have power to direct payment of part of it to the divorced spouse. Detailed recommendations were made for taking account of the complexities produced by SERPS.

The Pensions Management Institute considered the important benefit of lump sums payable on the death of a spouse before retirement. The amount is often substantial and can be up to four times the annual salary. Because trustees have discretion to choose to whom the sum should be payable and because it ceases if a member leaves a scheme, the PMI did not make radical recommendations. But it did recommend that the court should have power to require the maintenance payer to take out a life insurance policy to secure the maintenance. Such provisions are now frequently negotiated, but without the sanction of court power it is not possible to ensure such provision unless there is co-operation. The PMI also recommended that if the life of a spouse was not an insurable risk the court should have the power to require the divorced spouse to be included in the category of people who would benefit from death in service. The recommendations of the Pensions Management Institute have been set out at some length so that readers can have an idea of the variety of possibilities which could be legislated for. However, as mentioned earlier the Pensions Act 1995 has made some changes by importing into the Matrimonial Causes Act 1973 three new sub-sections.

The effect of the changes may be limited, and it is not yet known when they will take effect but their application will be affected by the as yet unpublished regulations the government will issue. The publicity given to the issue of pensions on divorce by the organisation Fair Shares (see p. 223), by the decision of the House of Lords in the case of *Brooks* (1995 2 FLR 13, HL) and the new law have made it certain for the future that pensions as an asset will not be ignored.

How much *Brooks* and the Pensions Act changes will affect decisions is problematic. The *Brooks* case will have application in a limited number of cases. It decided that the husband's post-marriage pension scheme which provided benefits for a group of people on his death, including a wife, was an arrangement which the court can vary as a post-nuptial (post-marriage) settlement under the Matrimonial Causes Act 1973 (Section 24) and it varied the scheme so that provision was made for the ex-wife. The court emphasised that it would not vary a scheme which involved a risk to the rights of third parties. In those circumstances the court would look at other non-pension asssets to compensate the wife.

Under the new Pensions Act the court has the duty to examine pension provision and has the power to earmark for the wife a proportion of the pension payable on the retirement of the husband, and vice versa. An order can be directed to the trustees of a pension fund and can require the husband with pension rights to commute the whole or part of his pension benefits. When a lump sum order is made the trustees can be ordered to pay it to the husband or can require him to nominate his ex-wife for receipt of a lump sum.

In cases where pensions are an important asset, wives (because it will usually be wives rather than husbands) will probably now wish to adjourn their ancillary relief applications until after the new regulations are published, because the retrospective position is not clear. Conversely, husbands will want their cases to be dealt with under the present law.

Another legislative change of relevance is the Finance Act 1995 Section 58 and Schedule 11. Personal pension holders can defer purchasing an annuity, that is to say their pension income, until the age of 75. However, they can draw some income in the meantime. Part of the fund can be taken by a wife or dependants subject to an income tax charge of 35 per cent, but payment of part of the policy does fall into the policy holder's estate and could be subject to inheritance tax.

The benefits of the new Pension Act provisions may be limited. For them to apply, the husband must survive to retirement age. It is already the case that a wife may obtain a nominal maintenance order which will enable her to apply for increased provision on her husband's retirement. This, like the new earmarking provisions, will run counter to the clean-break principle, because there will be no clean break if maintenance continues indefinitely. However, one must always bear in mind the possibility that a former husband may become unemployed or take early retirement.

What follows is of relevance to the present situation and is unlikely to be material when the Pension Act regulations are published.

In the course of a career the husband may be both employed and self-employed and may have arrangements in an occupational scheme as well as self-employed arrangements. The self-employed arrangements mentioned above usually make no provision for payment of benefit to a dependant unless a positive step is taken by the petitioner before the pension becomes payable. The benefit of a salaried scheme is the 'death in service' provision but it has to be recalled that the expression of wish in relation to the dependants to whom it should be paid, while usually followed by the trustees may not be followed if the trustees think the pension should be disbursed otherwise. They have complete discretion in the matter as the law stands at present. The pension, or regular payments for a widow or dependants when a spouse dies before retirement, are similar to those for a widow when death occurs after retirement. The beneficiary is usually a widow and not an ex-wife. The pension benefit may be a lump sum with a balance as pension, and a widow's pension may be up to two-thirds of the sum which the deceased would have received.

It is vital to obtain the necessary information about particular schemes. Parties involved in divorces will want to obtain detailed information about the pensions of their spouses in cases where the loss of pension may be a significant factor. To obtain this information a financial questionnaire is served on the prospective pensioner. This should include a question seeking a statement of the anticipated benefits on retirement and details of death in service provision. The Occupational Pension Schemes (Disclosure of Information) Regulations 1986 (Statutory Instrument 1986 no. 1046) obliges pension trustees to provide this information so that enquiry can be made of them directly. The regulations can be obtained from HMSO (address on p. 223). The Law Society recommends that a questionnaire be served on the solicitors acting for the future pensioner in the form set out in Appendix 4, p. 169. It may be necessary that the information be given to an actuary with instructions to estimate the potential loss to the wife that would ensue from divorce.

In the present state of the law the wife has limited options available where the value of the pension she is likely to lose is considerable. First, she can petition for judicial separation instead of divorce so that she remains married while still being able to get a financial settlement. The financial settlement will, however, not be final because the marriage has not been dissolved. Secondly, if she is the respondent to a divorce based on the fact that the parties have been separated for five years she may defend the petition on the basis of the grave financial hardship she would suffer if the marriage were dissolved; this approach may encourage her husband to make life insurance arrangements to compensate her. Such a wife will want to ensure that the periodical payments continue to be paid, and if they can be secured on an asset of the husband those payments will continue after his death. It follows that if the wife receives periodical payments there will be no dismissal of her rights against her husband's estate, because she will remain a dependant. She or her solicitor may be able to negotiate as part of a settlement the husband's agreement to nominate her to receive his death in service benefit, or a proportion of it. If this happens the husband should agree not to revoke the nomination later, and give the wife authority to enable her to check with the trustees from time to time to make sure no change has been effected.

Some pension schemes already allow pension benefits to an ex-wife. The Police Pension Scheme enables one-third of the pension to be allocated for a former wife or dependant. It is important to establish through the questionnaire under Rule 2.63 of the Family Proceedings Rules 1991 whether this exists in each case.

If an agreement is made on the proportion of lump sum which a wife will receive from the death in service provision, the question of life insurance is not so important. Replacement insurance to cover the benefits a wife would lose, including the loss of death in service benefit, is exceedingly expensive, 'demonstrating', as one author puts it, 'as a matter of evidence the real benefits the wife has lost'. The policy to be taken out is to provide, with the lump sum the ex-wife will receive, an additional sum at normal retirement date which can be used together with a lump sum proportion to provide an annuity for her (or other investment, dependent on prevailing market conditions at the time). If an insurance policy is taken out the wife's periodical payments sum should be increased to enable her to pay the premium.

The court can be asked to award a deferred lump sum whose amount will be based on the lump sum payable to the pensioner on retirement when the pension becomes payable. The lump sum element cannot be more than 25 per cent of the value of the pension fund. Another possibility is for the husband to add to the value of the wife's own pension. She may not have used her complete pension allowance in making her own annual contributions and may be able to make additional voluntary contributions for the years she has been in employment. It will be of great assistance to her if the husband can by a lump sum payment help her to make those additional voluntary contributions. What has been said in relation to husbands and wives applies *mutatis mutandis* if the wife has better pension arrangments than the husband.

Where there is sufficient capital to provide a clean break there will be no separate additional provision for a lump sum to reflect the prospective loss of widow's pension. In *Bee* v. *Bee* (1989 1 FLR 119) this was the view taken by the judge when awarding the wife a sum to enable her to purchase a home which in later years would be larger than her needs; she could sell this in exchange for a smaller property later on. The value of a lost pension can be calculated on the basis of the husband's expected pension. A formula has been devised to make the calculation. It is based on the cost, at the husband's normal retirement date, of buying a widow's pension and takes into account the age difference between them and the possibility that pensions will increase at variable rates. The method is demonstrated in the tables published in *At a Glance*, a valuable booklet published by the Family Law Bar Association. A 1987 case (*Duxbury* v. *Duxbury* 1987 1 FLR 10) provided that the payments the husband would make should be converted into a lump sum to meet the wife's future reasonable requirements in relation to both capital and income. Subsequent cases have shown that the calculations are not to be slavishly followed. A significant difference to be noted is that in cases involving larger sums of capital the money to be made available to a wife, which takes account of the loss of future income, is to meet the rather more generous standards of the demands of 'reasonable requirements' than the more basic ones of 'needs' to be assessed in cases involving less money.

Chapter 13

Foreign element

An increasing number of marriages occur between people one or both of whom live or have their permanent homes outside of England and Wales or who move to their original country if the marriage breaks down. If either of the parents or indeed a child is ordinarily resident outside the jurisdiction the Child Support Act will not apply to questions concerning the maintenance of the children. If either or both of them, on the breakdown of a marriage, wish to take proceedings in the jurisdiction of the courts in England and Wales they can institute divorce proceedings provided one of them has been ordinarily resident within the jurisdiction for more than one year or is domiciled here.

If the marriage took place abroad the proof of its validity is required by production of the original marriage certificate, as it is in cases where the marriage took place in England or Wales. If the marriage certificate is in a foreign language it should be translated by someone competent to do so and the translation should be filed with the certificate and the particulars of the translator's qualification.

Where there is a choice of jurisdiction as to where the proceedings should be taken, a petitioner should take advice as to which jurisdiction it would be better to invoke. For instance if a party living in Scotland does not wish his recent inheritance to be brought into account as part of his resources he may prefer to petition in Scotland although his wife is living in England. It may be possible for a financial application to be brought in England and Wales even if a divorce has taken place abroad, but the advantage may be with the court where the divorce was initiated.

Before 1984, if a husband obtained a foreign divorce a wife could make no financial claim because claims under the Matrimonial Causes Act 1973 can be made only when a decree has been pronounced in a court in England and Wales. The position was changed by the Matrimonial and Family Proceedings Act 1984 Part iii) under which, with the leave of the court, an applicant can pursue a financial claim here even if the decree has been pronounced abroad. To obtain leave an application can be made without serving the other party (an ex-parte application) on an originating summons (form M25) supported by an affidavit. Remarriage by either party is a bar to a claim and the applicant must satisfy the court that he or she has substantial grounds for an application. However, in one case (Z v. Z (Financial Provision. Overseas Divorce 1992 2 FLR 291)) the judge did not grant the wife's application to make a claim. The reasons were that she was already worth £850,000 and since her husband had £2 million worth of assets the court considered there were no substantial grounds for the application. Furthermore, the wife had committed adultery and deceived the court as to the extent of her own assets.

It has also been said by the Court of Appeal in that the change in the law in 1984 was not made to enable the English courts to review decisions made by foreign courts. In a recent decision giving an English ex-wife of an Italian leave to pursue an application here, the Court of Appeal made a distinction between cases where an applicant was 'forum shopping', that is pursuing a claim in the court of the state which might be most favourable to the claim, and those where a wife's only order, as in this case, was for maintenance pending suit in a magistrates' court in England. Delay will be a material factor: in this case the court attributed it to the fact that the wife's solicitors 'did not get the case off the ground' and the wife was therefore not responsible for the delay (*Lamagni* v. *Lamagni* 1995 2 FLR, CA).

The next problem facing an applicant is to satisfy the court that at the time of the foreign divorce either party was domiciled in England or Wales or can establish habitual residence there during the next 12 months before the hearing of the application or pronouncement of the decree. Either party must also have had a beneficial interest in property in England and Wales which was the matrimonial home. The court's decision will further depend upon whether or not it considers it appropriate for the English court to make the order. Considerations of relevance include the connection with England or Wales of the parties, the financial benefit to the applicant or any child of the family which might result from the proceedings and the utility of an order. If the only asset in question in England and Wales is a house the court can only deal with a lump sum claim and not periodical payments, but it can entertain claims under the Inheritance Act.

Property abroad can be dealt with by the court in England or Wales and removal of property to a foreign country cannot oust the jurisdiction of the English court. But if the foreign court is dealing with the matter the English court will not interfere.

Reference was been made at the end of Chapter 5 to the powers of the court to make Mareva injunctions to prevent the disposal of assets. Because the 1968 European Convention on Jurisdiction and the Enforcement of Judgments in Civil and Commercial Matters have the force of law here, Section 25 of the Civil Jurisdiction and Judgments Act 1982 gives power to the court to grant relief in England and Wales where proceedings have been taken in a contracting state. It seems that it can avail to get an injunction to enforce a claim for maintenance and lump sum. The same basis applies for relief here as if an application is made; the application has to have an arguable case, assets in the jurisdiction and a risk that they will be dissipated.

The enforcement abroad of maintenance orders made here is a very complex issue. It is reduced to clear essentials in the Law Society publication *The Enforcement of English Maintenance Orders Abroad* (1992). The first question the prospective applicant needs to consider is the availability of legal aid here or abroad. Certain European countries receive applications for legal aid from others, with the Legal Aid Board here acting as a postbox. Other information can be obtained from the Solicitors Family Law Association publication, *European Handbook*.

Whether a party abroad has assets to make enforcement worthwhile may be the critical question to be determined by enquiry agents. The Legal Practice Directorate Information Office can be asked about the employment of enquiry agents abroad. It is essential to obtain representation by solicitors familiar with the field and help can also be obtained from the Magistrates' Court Division of the Lord Chancellor's Department or the Children's Legal Centre (see pp. 223–4 for addresses and telephone numbers).

The vital distinction to be made, which affects decisions on the procedure to be followed, is between provisional orders and final orders. A provisional order is obtained after the prospective payer has left and it cannot be enforced unless confirmed by a foreign court. The final order is obtained before the payer leaves the country.

The legislation governing the procedures is contained in a number of different Acts of Parliament. There may be a choice of procedures to be followed and is important that professional guidance should be given as to which one is appropriate.

In the public mind the enforcement of English orders abroad is concerned more with the fate of children who may have been abducted by someone without the consent of 'a person connected with the child', that is a parent or guardian or person who has parental responsibility for the child. It is a criminal offence under the Child Abduction Act 1984 to remove a child under 16 from the United Kingdom. The courts have a procedure by which they inform the police of the imminent unlawful removal of a child. The procedure is set out in a Practice Direction made in 1986 (1 AE 983) and it is also described in a Home Office Circular no. 21/1986.

The civil law on the subject is governed by the Child Abduction and Custody Act 1985, Part I of which gives the effect to the Hague Convention of 1980 on the Civil Aspects of International Child Abduction. This provides for the expeditious return of children to the country where they have habitual residence if they have been wrongly removed by a contracting state. Part II of the Act gives effect to the European Convention of 1980 on recognition and enforcement of decisions concerning custody of children and on restoration of custody of children.

Under Article 3 of the Hague Convention the removal of a child is wrong where it is in breach of the custody rights attributed by law to the person with whom the child is habitually resident. Thus when a mother had interim custody in Ontario under an order which provided that the child was not to be removed from Ontario without leave of the court, and the mother brought the child to England in breach of this order, on the father's application in the English court an order was made for the return of the child to Ontario.

There is concern to ensure that where an order for a return is made it must be effected within six weeks or the central authority in the contracting state (in this country the Lord Chancellor's Department) can require reasons for the delay. But Article 13 of the Convention prevents the return if the person having custody did not exercise his or her rights or acquiesced in the removal of the child. In the case of *re S* 1994 (*The Times*, 16 February 1994 and *Independent*, 25 February 1994) the Court of Appeal held that bad advice given to a father did not mean he acquiesced in the child's removal. The mother had brought three children from —— to England and the father had been wrongly advised about the cost of bringing proceedings for their return to —— under the 1985 Act. When he discovered that he would get legal aid he took proceedings and the Court of Appeal upheld that there was no acquiescence in the decision. Even if there had been acquiescence the father might have succeeded unless the mother could use Article 13 of the Convention.

Article 13 of the Convention provides that a child will not be returned to the country where he or she is habitually resident if there is grave risk that the child would be exposed to physical or psychological harm or be placed in an intolerable situation. It is, however, clear that if the removal was wrongful the court must order the return of a child unless such a grave risk is apparent. If the risk and/or wishes of the child can be investigated in the country where he or she habitually resides, the child's removal will be ordered. In England and Wales an application under the Hague Convention and the European Convention is governed by the provisions of the Family Proceedings Rules Part 6. It is made by an originating summons in which there should be set out the necessary information about the child or children and their parents or guardians, and particulars of any proceedings must be accompanied by relevant documentation. The summons has to be acknowledged within seven days after it has been served and affidavit evidence can be filed by each party. The hearing of the original summons can be adjourned for a period on each occasion not exceeding 21 days.

Chapter 14

Mediation

This is the name given to the process intended to enable couples themselves to decide, subject to their right to independent legal advice, to resolve or minimise the issues in dispute between them.

In December 1993 the government issued a consultative Green Paper on divorce reform and mediation. This was followed in 1995 by a White Paper. These documents were precursors of the present Family Law Bill whose provisions were discussed in the Introduction. The consultation papers reviewed the present system without referring to the obligation solicitors have to try and reach a settlement of disputed matters. The papers considered recommendations made by the Law Commission in its discussion paper published in 1988, *Facing the Future*, and its final report, *The Grounds for Divorce* (1990).

The Family Law Bill envisages divorce on the basis of a divorce order or a separation order after a period of one year for reflection and consideration. The year is to begin when a statement of breakdown has been filed with the court and that step cannot take place until the person concerned has attended a public information session. The obligation to attend a public information session applies before any party makes an application to the court relating to a child of the family or property or financial matters. The bill provides that power for the court after it has received the statement of marital breakdown to direct the parties to attend a meeting explaining mediation and provide them with an opportunity to make use of mediation.

In Part 2 of the Family Law Bill provision is made for mediation in family matters but the Legal Aid Board's provision of mediation for persons who may be financially eligible makes it plain that the circumstances in which mediation is to be provided will be set out in regulations. It also provides that mediation will be granted only if it appears to a mediator that mediation is suitable. It appears that the Legal Aid Board will be able to decide whether someone should be permitted to have legal aid for representation in the courts if they have agreed to mediation except in circumstances which have yet to be prescribed. This then is the uncertain background against which mediation as it is now practised needs to be considered.

Mediation organisations are anxious to ensure that the government provides funding for mediation so that it is universally available. Such funding seems unlikely unless it is diverted from the money currently used to fund legal aid. There is particular concern about the imbalance which would be created between a couple who mediate where one has the means to obtain prior legal advice and the other has had none or has no possibility of obtaining any.

The conciliation movement developed from a conciliation scheme in relation to disputes concerning children in Bristol County Court from 1975. Since then conciliation has developed in relation to children so that all of the 118 divorce courts try to resolve disputes concerning them by conciliation appointments where a district judge, the parties and their legal advisers and a welfare officer are present. The issues discussed are contact and residence disputes affecting children. The purpose of the conciliation appointment is to establish whether there is any possibility of agreeing on contact which is disputed or on the residence. Appointments are given after one party has filed a statement under the Children Act. The discussions which take place are relatively informal compared with court procedure and the parties have an opportunity to discuss the matter separately with the welfare officer. In the Principal Registry children over the age of 9 are also brought to the court so that they can be seen in a separate room by a welfare officer. Where there is no agreement the district judge is able to make an order providing directions for the way in which the application should be dealt with.

There have been numerous discussions about the meanings of conciliation and mediation. The *Oxford English Dictionary* definition of conciliate is 'to gain goodwill etc. by acts which induce friendly feeling', or to reconcile. To mediate, on the other hand, is to act as 'an intermediary to intervene for the purpose of reconciling and to settle a dispute by mediation'.

The new edition of the Law Society's *Guide to the Professional*

Conduct of Solicitors published in 1995 permits solicitors who have hitherto been instructed by one party to offer mediation as part of their practice without necessarily having any mediation training or a code of practice to which to adhere. Solicitors have for some years been permitted to act as lawyer mediators for the Family Mediators Association which trains and accredits them, monitors their practice and provides continuing training. As mediators for the Family Mediators Association solicitors have to have separate insurance arrangements.

Many forms of mediation are conducted away from the courts. The Family Mediators Association and National Family Mediation (formerly National Association of Family Mediation and Conciliation Services) were mentioned in Chapter 2. The former has between 300 and 400 mediators, half of whom are lawyers. The affiliated National Family Mediation has mediators who are appointed in a number of different ways following an aptitude test. National Family Mediation is developing comprehensive mediation on financial issues as well as child issues, and some of the mediators working for its affiliated services are lawyers. Both organisations agreed in February 1994 to work out a joint programme to lead to their merger.

Traditionally the mediation model employed by the Family Mediators Association (FMA) involves the couple, as well as a lawyer mediator and a family mediator, both of whom have undergone a training course; admission to this depends on the extent of their responsibility and experience in their respective fields. Satisfactory completion and assessment during training lead to admission to the FMA. While this book has been in production, NFM and FMA have formed the UK College of Family Mediators.

The mediation organisations recognise that it is not the purpose of mediation to promote reconciliation or rescue marriages. But if these options are possible for the couple the mediators may identify them more readily than the traditional process of legal advice to each partner separately. It is important to stress that both the lawyer and the family mediator (in the FMA model) offer impartial help. The solicitor acting as a mediator is not acting as a solicitor and is providing information, not advice. Neither mediator is making a judgement. All correspondence and information are to be shared with both parties unless there is a telephone number or address which should not be disclosed. Full financial disclosure is required and this information is obtained on an open basis so that although the discussions are legally privileged the information cannot be. Of course the matters discussed in mediation can be discussed by each party with his or her own legal adviser, from whom advice may have been obtained before the mediation began and to whom reference may be made from time to time by the parties.

The prospect for a man or a woman contemplating divorce or seeing a solicitor is difficult but the suggestion that both of them should face each other in mediation to discuss differences and possible agreement face to face may be yet more daunting. Some clients feel happier if they have already consulted a solicitor before mediation. Some prefer to deal with mediators whom they know are obliged to be impartial, however stressful the encounter may be initially. Many broach the issue of divorce after consulting Relate or counsellors of one of the other organisations listed on pp. 223–4.

Before a couple meet mediators of the FMA each receives a letter setting out the principles on which the mediators work and their terms of reference. Each partner is required to sign an agreement to the terms. A further letter sets out the charges. Charging rates vary. Couples have sessions of one and a half hours and they pay for time spent by the mediators for written work done in between sessions at a rate pro rata to the charging rate. Each partner is sent a referral form, initially to elicit essential biographical information including particulars of the children's age, education, special needs and living arrangements. Some preliminary financial information is also sought on a short form.

The agenda for the first session is likely to be the present state of the marriage or relationship and the decisions or issues to be settled taking account of the needs of each party and the children involved.

The format of mediation meetings is informal and first names are generally used between the mediators and their clients. The emphasis is on forward-looking discussion rather than on analysis of the breakdown which concentrates on the past; this does not exclude discussion of the past but rather emphasises the need to plan solutions. The second session is preceded by completion by each party of a very detailed financial questionnaire. The number of sessions in the course of which terms of settlement may be worked out is between three and six. If proposals are made which can be agreed they will be set out in a summary prepared by the mediators. The agreement is 'without prejudice'. It is fundamentally important that clients should obtain independent advice before entering into a legally binding agreement. Whether agreement is finally reached or not, the disclosure of financial information, and often other information verified by the necessary documentation, can save solicitors time and the clients legal costs. The Family Law Bill, incredibly, makes no provision for the courts to approve agreed settlements. The implications for the professional liability of mediators have not, it seems, been considered by the parliamentary draftsman.

In services affiliated to National Family Mediation, mediation is undertaken by one mediator or by two working as co-mediators from a wide range of backgrounds. There is no formal requirement as to professional qualifications and length of experience, but in practice a majority have a social work or counselling background. In some circumstances a lawyer co-mediator is brought in at different stages. Historically, NFM provided help to couples in an attempt to resolve disputes concerning children but it now offers a variety of comprehensive mediation models. The Family Mediators Association and National Family Mediation shared a joint code of practice before their resolution to merge in the UK College of Family Mediators late in 1995.

Since the formation of the Solicitors Family Law Association in 1982 more family solicitors have adopted an approach to settlement of disputes which, since the decision in the case of *Evans* v. *Evans* 1990, has been required of all solicitors (see Appendix 2).

If the Family Law Bill becomes law as drafted the opportunities for independent legal advice and representation on settlement proposals may be limited. The circumstances in which independent legal advice is essential are many. For example it may have been proposed at mediation to sell the matrimonial home and give two-thirds of the proceeds to the wife, with whom the young children will live in a different house with her new partner. The husband seeking his solicitor's advice may be advised that a lower proportion would be justified, given that the wife is to remarry, because her needs and those of the children could be met by a lower proportion even if it were more than 50 per cent of the proceeds. An experienced solicitor, however, will be aware of the goodwill value of a settlement which may be more generous than the court might award and may advise that the proposals should not be changed. All depends on the individual circumstances and property values. Conversely, a wife may propose at mediation to accept less capital than her solicitor considers she would get because her husband is embarking on a new business venture from which she does not wish to discourage him. Mediators and the parties' own legal advisers need to explore how the wife intends to support herself and whether the payment of capital is intended to provide a clean break so that no further claims can be made in the future, or whether there is the prospect of maintenance claims being retained in case a wife should be unable to earn as much as she expects. If the difference between what a solicitor considers appropriate to be offered or accepted in mediation is a sum such as about £5,000, careful thought should given to whether it would be worth litigating in order to get more, or possibly less. The costs of litigation cannot be known in advance and it involves the risk that one party might have to pay a high proportion of the other's costs.

The findings of a number of research projects show that the benefits of mediation include reduced conflict and bitterness. The focus on parental co-operation and the needs of children and the flexibility of the process, which can be adapted to the parties' time scale and needs rather than the courts' timetable, the facilitation of dialogue and decision making enable both parties to feel in charge of the outcome. The avoidance of unnecessary correspondence and litigation, with all the stress and delays involved, cannot be too strongly emphasised. Properly resourced mediation attended by couples who are willing to undergo the process may well result in a saving to the taxpayer of the costs involved in the litigation route.

However, some cautionary notes about the benefits of mediation must be sounded. Some American research has suggested that no study of mediation has demonstrated a better outcome for children from mediation than litigation ('Long-term effects of divorce mediation in a field study of Child Custody Dispute Resolution', submitted to the *American Journal of Ortho-Psychiatry* in 1995). Secondly, mediation is inappropriate unless it is voluntary and will always be inappropriate if there has been violence or if there is need for protective litigation, such as steps to protect a family from violence. The mediation process can also be undermined by an imbalance between the parties unless this is successfully counteracted by the mediators. Some imbalances are too great to be counteracted and it would be an inappropriate use of public resources to insist that there be forced mediation as a precondition of legal aid for legal representation in relation to financial or children matters. Finally, and most importantly, independent legal advice on any without prejudice agreement is essential.

Chapter 15

The mechanics of settlement

Vigorous litigation and the most civilised negotiations without litigation end, if pursued, in a court order. The order will be made in the teeth of opposition at the end of proceedings if the former course is pursued, and with a consent order if the latter. In between are many cases which settle at some point in the litigation.

There is a point in negotiations where delay on one party's side may have so prolonged the tension, and increased the costs, that an application for ancillary relief should be made to the court for it to determine the matter. The fact that proceedings have been instituted should be a trigger to more purposeful negotiations. External events may complicate or facilitate settlement prospects. A child may leave university and get a job. One of the parties may get a better job or lose one. The housing market in the area may change with the advent of a new firm or the disappearance of another. One party may develop a new relationship.

Where a case has been contested and the district judge hears it, judgment is usually delivered after both parties have given their evidence and been cross-examined and final speeches have been delivered by their solicitors or barristers. In a complex matter the decision may be given at the end of the hearing and the reasons given in a judgment later.

The judgment will recount the history of the marriage and the way in which the financial situation of the parties reached the present circumstances. Where issues have been in dispute the judge makes findings of fact on them. He or she may say that the explanation given for the disappearance of a sum of money from an account is unacceptable and the judge may, as he or she is entitled to do in a case of inadequate disclosure, draw adverse inferences from the evidence given. For example, the judge may say that although the husband swears that his earnings are £40,000 the evidence of his lifestyle compels a different conclusion; if it is a maintenance case the judge may order what he or she considers to be a realistic amount for the husband to pay if the wife needs it.

There may have been conflicting evidence about the value of an asset such as the matrimonial home. The judge will indicate which value he or she accepts as the basis for the order at the conclusion of the judgment.

The order is often for the solicitors or barristers to draft. In a case where all matters are agreed and there is no hearing, the solicitor for one party drafts an order, the other amending it if necessary, and both sign it. Sometimes both parties sign it also. If no affidavits have been filed because the parties have not litigated, an application for financial relief has to be filed by the respondent (the petitioner's prayer for relief, it will be recalled, is in the petition). The application will be headed 'for dismissal purposes only' and it will not be necessary to pay a fee of £20 on it as it would (unless a litigant is legally aided) when an application is issued to initiate financial proceedings. The other document to be completed and signed by or on behalf of each party is the statement of means, which contains the briefest summary of income and assets prior to the agreed division. It also requires each party to state whether or not they are cohabiting or remarrying or intend to do so.

Even when a couple have successfully negotiated a settlement it is desirable that they should receive independent legal advice, as this book has continually emphasised. It is essential to ensure that the terms of the consent order are embodied in a form acceptable to the judge who seals them. A consent order may be by agreement but it is an order of the court. It is crucially important that it should be phrased clearly and that if claims of any kind are to be dismissed the possibility of their being advised in future must be excluded. Hence the citing of all the legislation which is relevant in a case where maintenance and capital claims are to be dismissed. The relevant sections of the Matrimonial Causes Act 1973 and the Married Women's Property Act 1882 are referred to and the parties' claims under the Inheritance (Provision for Family and Dependants) Act will be dismissed as part of the order.

Many solicitors draft orders based on precedents prepared by the Solicitors Family Law Association which, although they do not have the official approval of the Principal Registry or any other divorce county court, have been drafted after discussions with the Association of County Court district judges and representatives of the Principal Registry.

The preliminary parts of an order recite what has occurred and the agreements reached. In a case where maintenance and capital claims are to be dismissed the preliminary first paragraph will state that the agreement is made on the basis that the provision made in the order is accepted in full and final settlement of all claims which the parties have against each other so that there will be no further claims by either of them when the terms of the order have been complied with. If it has been agreed that a property is to be sold it will be recited that it is to be placed on the market with agreed agents at a particular price, or at a price which the agents advise, and provision may be made for the firm of solicitors who are to be instructed to act on the sale.

Some categories of action cannot be ordered by the court but may have been agreed by the parties. It is nearly always undesirable to litigate about the contents of a house and most couples will try to agree between them what items each should have from it, it being often the case that the parent with whom the children live will have more of the furniture. It is sensible to record in the order that contents have been divided by agreement between the parties. If there is any question of uncertainty a schedule of the items taken by each party can be annexed to the order. Matters such as the discharge of an overdraft should be the subject of an undertaking. Another example where an undertaking should be given is a case where a husband agrees to nominate his death in service benefit or a proportion of it for the other spouse and agrees to ensure that the other has a right to inspect the nomination periodically. There may be an undertaking to take out a policy of insurance to cover maintenance or school fees and the actual order can provide that the payer will maintain the premiums on the policy. An undertaking is a solemn promise to the court and if it is not adhered to can be the subject of enforcement proceedings.

The actual order follows the recited agreement and undertakings. It may provide for the transfer of the matrimonial home to one party and the payment of a capital sum to a husband or wife who is making the transfer. It contains the provisions for maintenance for the wife, or husband, if appropriate, and for the children if agreed. Agreed payment of maintenance to a child is expressed to be payable to the wife for the children so that the relatively small amount of tax relief still available is obtained for the payer. Where a lump sum of capital is awarded it will be provided, as with the provision for transfer of a property, that it be made on or within a certain period of time. Only one lump sum can be awarded but that may be paid in instalments, as will be necessary when the entire sum cannot be raised at once, or when the payer is certain at a future date to receive a sum of money from which the further instalment is to be paid.

Maintenance may be dismissed by the order, or if the circumstances require it a nominal order may be made. This would enable a former wife to make claims in the future if she is unable to work. When continuing maintenance is ordered it may be provided that it will be reviewed in accordance with the Retail Price Index; but if circumstances warrant it an application for variation may be made when either party's circumstances justify it, as may be the case where one party loses a job or is forced to take a lower-paid job or has a significant promotion.

If maintenance is ordered to be paid, but for a limited period such as three years and is then to be dismissed, it has been held in a recent decision (*Richardson* v. *Richardson* 1994 1 FLR 286) that a wife was entitled to apply during the period for variation of the periodical payments. The reason was that the Matrimonial and Family Proceedings Act 1984 conferred on the courts two distinct powers, one to dismiss the right to maintenance and the other to prevent further applications. The right to apply for maintenance pending a clean break remained unless the order contained a direction that no application could be made to extend the payments.

If no further claim of capital or maintenance is to be made, those rights will be dismissed. There may be an order for costs or it may be limited to a specific and agreed contribution or there may be no order as to costs. It is customary and sensible to have a final provision called 'liberty to apply as to the implementation of the terms of this order'. There may be disagreement as to what a particular term means and such issues can be referred back to the district judge for clarification or determination if the drafting of the words has left the matter in doubt.

A transfer of property or a lump sum order which is final cannot be varied. There will, however, be cases when a fact of financial relevance becomes known to one party after the order is made. If the fact is something which was concealed when disclosure was made and the effect might have altered the terms of the order an application can be made to set the order aside. An order can be set aside on the basis of non-disclosure and fraud and, less commonly, fresh evidence (*Barder* v. *Barder* 1988 AC 20 where a wife's death after the transfer was made meant there was no reason for the transfer), lack of consent and bad legal advice.

One case of non-disclosure where an order was subsequently set aside concerned the failure of a husband to disclose that he was selling shares in his company (*Vicary* 1992 2 FLR).

It may happen that, several months after a final order, a woman marries a man whom she knew before the order was made, and whom, at the time she completed the financial statement, she says she had no intention of marrying or cohabiting with. Her former husband may wish to set aside the order on the basis that if the court had known of her intention the size of her capital award would not have been as great; much will depend upon her evidence (*Prow* v. *Brown* 1983 4 FLR 352).

Or it may be that an asset is sold shortly after the order is made for a far greater figure than the valuation given to it for the purposes of settlement or trial (see *Allsop* v. *Allsop* 1980 11 FLR 18, CA). Or the court's decision may have been based on a valuation which is later shown to have been excessive. In a 1992 case (*Heard* v. *Heard* Court of Appeal 1995 1 FLR) where the wife's valuation of the matrimonial home indicated that it had an equity of £55,000, and the husband had obtained no valuation, the court ordered that the property be sold and £16,000 be paid to the wife so that the husband could rehouse himself with the balance. After the husband had unsuccessfully tried to borrow £16,000 on the security of the property and then to sell it, he tried to appeal the court's decision out of time. The only offers he had received were £30,000 and £33,000. The court refused leave and the husband appealed to the Court of Appeal, where he succeeded in obtaining leave. The Court of Appeal held that the husband was not to be seriously criticised for the delay because he had tried to raise money in order to avoid a sale and it was clear that the basis for the original order had radically changed. The case was sent to the county court for it to hear the appeal.

In another 1992 case the district judge made orders for the periodical payments for a wife and two children and for the wife to have a share in the matrimonial home. Subsequently, the husband's income and capital position improved dramatically following the rise in the share value in his company. When the wife failed in her application for leave to appeal out of time she applied for a variation of the maintenance orders and received an increase for herself of £15,000 per annum to £35,000 and a doubling of each child's maintenance from £4,200 per annum to £8,500 per annum. The payments were backdated to the date when the district judge had made the orders two years before. The husband appealed to the Court of Appeal unsuccessfully.

Before an appeal is launched it will always be necessary to take advice, to bear in mind that the court has very wide powers of discretion and to consider carefully the risks of an application, which may include the obligation to pay the costs of the other party if the applicant is unsuccessful.

Chapter 16

Death and taxes

Benjamin Franklin said that death and taxes were the only
certainties life offered. Divorcing couples have more reason than
others to plan for them because of the consequences which could
otherwise ensue.

Despite the fact that since 1938 the law has made what has
been described as 'a legislative incursion into the freedom of
testamentary disposition' it is better for anyone who has a child or
any property to make a will than not to do so.

Where there is a no will the law provides that the surviving
spouse inherits the entire estate of the deceased up to the amount
of £200,000 if there are no children. Otherwise, the surviving
spouse inherits the first £126,000 of the estate and the investment
income on half the remaining capital, while the children will
inherit the remaining half of the capital immediately and the rest
on the death of the surviving parent.

Whether a deceased who was domiciled in England or Wales
dies testate, that is having made a will, or intestate, the Inheritance
(Provision for Family and Dependants) Act of 1975 enables certain
people to make an application for financial provision from the
deceased's estate. The category of possible applicants includes the
wife or husband or former wife or husband who has not remarried,
a child of the deceased (who does not have to be a dependant (*re
Leach* 1985 2 AE 754), any person who was treated as a child of the
family in any marriage to which the deceased was a party and any
person not in the above category who was maintained wholly or
partly by the deceased. The matter for the court is whether the will
or the effect of the law on intestacy makes reasonable provision
for the applicant. The applicant has to make the claim within six
months of the grant of administration, if the deceased left no will,
or grant of probate if the deceased left a will.

The Law Reform (Succession) Act 1995 adds a new category to those who can apply for provision out of the estate of a deceased who dies on or after 1 January 1996: a person who 'during the whole of the period of two years ending immediately before the date when the deceased dies . . . was living (a) in the same household as the deceased, and (b) as the husband or wife of the deceased'. Dependency will no longer be a qualification. But if the applicant is adequately provided for, no provision will be made from the estate and the provision made will be limited to sums that are required for maintenance.

Under the present law, when an application is made by someone in one of the categories allowed by the Act the court has to consider the financial resources and needs of the applicant and those of any other applicant as well as the financial resources and financial needs of any beneficiary of the estate. The court has also to consider the obligations and responsibilities which the deceased had towards the applicant or towards any beneficiary, the size and nature of the net estate and any physical or mental disability of an applicant or of any beneficiary. Apart from the conduct of the applicant, another matter which may be relevant to the circumstances the court may also consider is what provision the applicant might have expected to receive if on the day the deceased died the marriage had ended not by death but by divorce. The difficulty in this approach is that with divorce both spouses remain alive but where death has occurred additional monies may be added to the available assets by way of insurance policies which mature on death and there may be liabilities such as inheritance tax. The success of a former wife or husband in any application will of course depend to some extent on his or her circumstances resulting from the death, for example where a periodical payments order ceased because the payer died.

An applicant wishing to argue that, within six years of death, the deceased, intending to defeat his or her claims in divorce proceedings, transferred property to another person at an undervalue can apply to the court for an order under Section 10(2) of the Inheritance (Provision for Family and Dependants) Act. If the applicant is successful the court orders the transfer of the property to the applicant after deduction of the inheritance tax which may have been borne by the recipient of the property. The sum must not exceed the value at the deceased's death of the property disposed of. In the case of *Dawkins* v. *Judd* (1986 2 FLR 60) the deceased sold the matrimonial home to his daughter in order to prevent an order being made for financial provision for his widow under the 1975 Act. The widow applied to the court and the daughter was ordered to pay a lump sum from the proceeds of sale of the house.

A testator cannot prevent an application being made by any potential applicant although he or she may wish to state in his or her will the reason why any provision made for a potential applicant is relatively small or why no provision is being made at all. It may be a good reason, such as the level of provision which was made by the court following divorce, or it may be that further provision has been made by an insurance policy which would not form part of the deceased's estate, or it may be because property has been transferred to the deceased during the testator's lifetime in order to safeguard the property from inheritance tax.

Divorcing couples will be concerned to ensure that where there is no question of continuing maintenance possible future claims against the estate of the other shall be agreed to be dismissed. Where there has been no agreed settlement and the financial applications have been decided after litigation, the court will make such provision part of the order if there is no continuing maintenance to a wife.

In the interval between the beginning of separation and the dissolution of the marriage couples may wish to make new wills. They will in any case take steps to try and ensure that joint properties such as bank and building society accounts are not closed without their authority. Where the matrimonial home or second home are owned on the basis of a joint tenancy the death of one of them means that the other will inherit. Either may wish to prevent this happening by creating a tenancy in common. This is done by serving a notice of severance on the other owner (see Appendix 1). Providing proof of service has been given to the Land Registry, a restriction is placed on the title to the property. This has the effect of preventing one spouse giving a receipt for the purchase price of the property. On the death of one spouse the property will be sold unless agreement can be reached on the terms on which the co-owner can purchase the share of the deceased.

If the property is unregistered land the notice of severance will be with the deeds and so should be seen by anyone proposing to lend money on the security of the property. A spouse who believes that, for example, the unregistered property he or she owns with his or her partner will be inherited by that partner and left to someone outside the family may wish to do what he or she can by preserving his/her share for the children. The spouse may wish to sever the joint tenancy and the way to protect the share for the children will be to register with the Land Registry a caution against the first registration of the property. This would prevent the other spouse if he or she survives from disposing of the property as he or she wished without providing for the share of the deceased because when unregistered property is sold it has now to be registered with the Land Registry.

The effect of the decree absolute on a will is to nullify any gift to a spouse or appointment as executor and a notice to this effect appears on the order making the decree nisi. The testator appointing an ex-spouse as an executor will make plain that he or she is a former husband or wife. Under the Law Reform (Succession) Act 1995 in the case of a death on or after 1 January 1996, divorce or annulment of marriage will be treated like death where a former spouse is appointed an executor or given an interest in property. Until then a gift or appointment merely lapses, that is to say it will be dealt with as if the testator was intestate. This was exemplified in a case in 1985 (*re Sinclair* 1985 FLR 965, CA): here the testator left his estate to his wife provided she survived for one month, but if she failed to survive him or predeceased him his estate was left to a charity. Before his death the testator divorced his wife, who survived him. As a result his estate was dealt with as if he had died without making a will. From the beginning of 1996 the effect of divorce on such a will will be to enable the charity to inherit.

Another change in the new Act is that the appointment of a guardian either by will or by some other written document is changed by divorce unless there is evidence that the appointment was intended to continue.

A more difficult problem can arise where, following divorce and remarriage, no will has been made. Where two people die in circumstances making it uncertain which survived longer it is presumed that the younger died later. In the case of a second marriage where a second wife is younger than her husband and both die intestate any children of the wife will inherit both estates. The children of the first marriage will of course be potential applicants under the Inheritance Act but the problems of litigation can be avoided or reduced by the preventive measure of each party making a will.

If the matrimonial home is transferred by a court order on divorce no stamp duty or other tax is payable on it nor is any tax payable in respect of a lump sum ordered to be transferred, although if a property has to be sold to pay a lump sum capital gains tax is payable on the sale of that property. If other property, such as a second home, is transferred capital gains tax may be payable when it is sold unless it is transferred in the financial year of separation or it falls within what is known as the Extra Statutory Concession D6. This deems that the spouse transferring the matrimonial home has continued in occupation of it provided he or she has not elected to treat any other property as his or her main residence.

Capital gains tax is calculated on the increase in value of an asset (whether it is an investment, a second home or other property) since 6 April 1982. If the property was acquired after that date the increase in value is calculated from the date of the acquisition. Against the increase in value of the property over the period the rate of inflation for the same time calculated according to the Retail Price Index can be offset, and so can the cost of improvements. Additionally, the first £6,300 of the increase in value is exempt. The tax payable on the excess is 25 per cent in the case of a standard rate taxpayer or 40 per cent in the case of a taxpayer whose income is sufficient to pay at the higher rate.

If an order is made under the Inheritance Act where a marriage has not been dissolved the disposition is exempt from inheritance tax (Section 18 Inheritance Tax Act 1984). Inheritance tax may be payable where the marriage has been dissolved but if there are no proceedings under the Inheritance Act or they are settled without an order, the sums may not attract inheritance tax. It is vital to obtain specialist advice on the problem.

Since 5 April 1990 there has been independent taxation of husband and wife. Before that date they submitted joint tax returns and were taxed together. Under the present system the husband has the single person's relief of £3,520 and the married couple's allowance of £1,720 unless his income is too low. There is a higher married couple's allowance of £2,145 for those over 65 and of £2,185 for those over 75.

The Finance Act 1988 made changes to the Income and Corporation Taxes Act of 1970 the effect of which was to make maintenance paid to a separated spouse payable gross and not to be taxed in the hands of the recipient. The payer qualifies for tax relief at 15 per cent on £1,720 only. Payments made to a spouse for the benefit of a child attract the same relief but the relief is only one amount of relief and the payments must be made under a court order or written agreement. Complex provisions apply in relation to orders made before the tax year 1988–89 but they are largely outside the scope of this book. It is important however, to emphasise that when maintenance orders made before 1988–89 are varied upwards the payer's tax relief will be restricted to the exact amount of relief he or she received under the old law: it will not be reduced to the narrow margin applicable to new orders.

In the post 1988–89 situation the effect is thus: if a husband pays maintenance of £5,000 per annum to his wife and £5,000 to the wife for his child, he only gets the same relief at the standard rate on £1,720 as he would if he paid maintenance to just one of them. The tax relief received by the payer is therefore worth £430 (25 per cent of £1,720). Because maintenance, unlike earnings, is not taxed there is no disincentive to work if work is available and the wife has the opportunity to do it. Where maintenance is paid at a lower level than the maximum income support allowances which are available from the Department of Social Security a wife may wish to increase maintenance. But she will not wish to put at risk the benefits which accompany income support, such as housing benefit and free school meals (see Chapter 10). Where maintenance is paid for the benefit of a child under a child maintenance assessment made by the Child Support Agency the same tax relief is available to the payer as under a court order for maintenance to be paid to a wife for the benefit of a child.

If maintenance is paid by an ex-spouse who dies and his or her estate continues to pay maintenance, for example if it were secured, it is probable that the payments are exempt from inheritance tax. Some payments from one spouse to another before or after divorce as well as lump sums paid to a child are exempt from inheritance tax as well as capital gains tax and income tax mentioned above.

Where a court makes an order to reverse a transfer of property or avoid a disposition, as Section 37 MCA 1973 describes it (see p. 35), and a transaction is set aside, the Inland Revenue treats the transfer of the property which is handed back as a 'disposal' for capital gains tax purposes. It is presumed to be transferred back at market value, and capital gains tax is levied on the market value. (Capital Gains Tax Act 1979 Section 29A). When the property is handed back following an order made under the Inheritance Act 1975 the property becomes part of a deceased's estate for inheritance tax purposes.

Reference was made earlier to the application of Section 17 of the Married Women's Property Act 1882 to obtaining a declaration of interest in property. The same section may benefit a spouse who has paid for a second home which is owned in joint names. If the court transfers the property under Section 24 of the Matrimonial Causes Act there may be capital gains tax to pay in respect of the half-share transferred. If the spouse applies under Section 17 for a declaration that she is entitled to it, it may be allowed on the basis that there is a presumption of resulting trust so that there will be no capital gains tax or inheritance tax because the husband's position would have been that he had been a trustee (someone owning his share for the benefit of his wife) and not a beneficial owner owning his share because he was entitled to it.

Where couples separate and one leaves the matrimonial home the question that arises is which one is entitled to MIRAS (mortgage interest relief at source) on the mortgage payments. If the mortgage was taken out before 6 April 1988, whichever spouse pays the interest gets the tax relief. If the husband leaves and pays it he cannot get interest relief on a mortgage for a new home so it is better to give maintenance to the wife for her to pay the mortgage. The problem arises if the question of benefit entitlement is relevant, because if the wife has housing benefit from the Department of Social Security there will be no question of MIRAS relief.

When spouses live together they have only one exemption. Exemption from capital gains tax for their residence is shared between them. The election as to which of two houses is the main residence operates retrospectively for up to two years. Thereafter, unless the Inland Revenue Extra Statutory Concession D6 (see p. 139 above) gives relief from capital gains, the tax will be payable.

The clean-break option often employed in the past is a method of giving a wife and family security in the matrimonial home but it is unlikely to be used as frequently in the future unless maintenance for children is agreed and likely to continue to be agreed and it is unlikely that the wife will ever be dependent on income support or family credit. The alternative to a clean break for the husband is a charge for his share of the matrimonial home or continued ownership on terms which enable him to realise his share when his wife cohabits permanently or remarries or when the youngest child ends full-time education. Such an outcome involves a risk of liability to capital gains tax on the difference between the value of the property at the date of the order and the amount realised on eventual sale subject to the deductions set out above. Liability would not arise if a specific amount was stated to be payable to the former husband on sale but that arrangement would not reflect any increase which might occur in the value of the house.

For example, if at the time of divorce in 1992 half the equity in the house was worth £20,000 and it was agreed that the former husband's share was one half, this proportion can be so referred to in the order dealing with financial matters. At the time of sale ten years later half the equity may be worth £25,000 and that will be the former husband's entitlement, with no liability to capital gains tax because the amount of increase does not attract it. If the share had been fixed at £20,000 the former husband would suffer. Conversely, if the equity had diminished to, say, £7,000 the former wife would suffer because the amount she would be obliged to pay her husband would remain fixed at £10,000.

Regulations passed under the 1991 Child Support Act do now permit an amendment to the formula in the few cases where it can be shown that there has been a capital settlement which benefits the children. There is also provision in the Child Support Act 1995 for departures from the formula in certain circumstances. Those circumstances are defined restrictively, in the draft regulations published in 1996 (see p. 000), but how they will work will not be apparent until they are applied nationally from the end of the year.

Chapter 17

Enforcement of court orders

The orders of the court would be meaningless without methods to ensure compliance with them. It would, however, be unrealistic to expect that even the most draconian methods can always be guaranteed to be effective.

The two kinds of enforcement with which this chapter is concerned are the enforcement of orders to do or not to do certain things; and financial orders for periodical payments, lump sums or costs. Enforcement of orders abroad was considered in Chapter 13.

In the first category are orders to answer questions put under Rule 2.63 of the Family Proceedings Rules 1991, that is to say those questions which are designed to elicit information and documents about a party's means. The reason for an application to the district judge for the questions to be answered is a respondent's failure to respond to those questions voluntarily. The district judge's order will provide for a response to the questions that he or she considers should be answered with a realistic time limit. If no replies are then forthcoming or are incomplete a further order may be sought for their immediate reply, coupled, perhaps, with an application that in default of an immediate response, the other party be debarred from further defending the case. At each stage the party applying for the order will seek to recover the costs of the applications.

A penal notice may also be sought at this stage. This is a notice warning the other party that he or she may face committal to prison if the order is not obeyed. The order endorsed with this notice has to be served personally on the respondent if an application is to be made to the court to commit him or her to prison for breach of the order when 28 days have expired if the order has not been complied with.

Committal to prison is a punishment for contempt of court, that is to say disobeying a court order, whether it is an order to answer questions, to refrain from violence or to pay money. Since committal does not secure the information required nor produce the money ordered to be paid nor regulate behaviour as provided by an injunction made by the court it is very much a last resort.

Where one party to proceedings refuses to comply with an order for a transfer of property such as the matrimonial home the other can apply to the court for an order that it may be executed by an officer of the court. This delays the transfer and causes more costs to be incurred which the party in contempt will no doubt try to avoid paying. The method of enforcement of that order will be described below.

The choice of the method of enforcing a money order depends on the kind of order which was made and the amount of money involved. The Maintenance Orders Act 1958 provided two new methods of enforcing orders, one by registering High Court orders in the magistrates' court and vice versa, and the other by attaching the earnings of the debtor. Now the High Court, the Principal Registry and divorce county courts have powers to enforce orders.

Arrears of maintenance overdue for more than one year can only be enforced with leave of the court. Other orders must be enforced within six years. The order to be enforced should be served personally on the debtor and endorsed with a penal notice. If a debtor dies, the costs when taxed can be claimed against his or her estate. Likewise when a creditor dies his or her personal representatives or executors can claim costs for the estate.

Enforcement of the obligation of an employed person to pay maintenance can perhaps most usefully be achieved by attachment of earnings proceedings now governed by the Attachment of Earnings Act 1971. The application can be made to the magistrates' court in an order that can be enforced there, to a county court or the High Court. For an order to be made one or more payments must be due and 15 days must have expired since the order.

An order will not be made if it appears that failure to pay was not due to 'wilful refusal or wilful neglect'. If the debtor does not attend the court hearing fixed for the application the hearing may be adjourned for up to 14 days. Imprisonment is the risk if there is a further failure to appear. Alternatively, an order for commitment to prison may be suspended until the debtor fails to appear on a further occasion.

The debtor's employer is obliged to comply with an attachment of earnings order. The employer will not incur liability until seven days after service of the order. An explanatory booklet from the Home Office explains how an order operates (*Attachment of Earnings Explanatory Booklet for Employers*). The order states what will be the normal deduction rate and which protected earning rates apply, and it must contain enough information to identify the debtor. The normal deduction rate is the amount that the court thinks it reasonable (after payment of tax) to deduct to pay maintenance and arrears of maintenance within a reasonable period. The protected earning rate is the rate below which earnings should not be reduced. It is based on income support allowances. Employers can deduct collection costs according to the Attachment of Earnings (Employment Deduction) Order 1991. Provision is made for reducing the amount deducted, for example when the arrears are paid off so only the current maintenance is thereafter deducted.

The court may discharge an order if an employer no longer employs the debtor or the order ceases to have effect, or the order may be varied when it is redirected to a newer employer. The court which makes the order is the one which made the maintenance order unless the maintenance order was made in a county court and is registered in a magistrates' court where it can then be enforced.

In practice an application for an attachment of earnings order is made in the court which made the maintenance order, but Part 1 of the Maintenance Orders Act 1958 enables orders to be registered in the magistrates' court where an application for an attachment of earnings order is made by a complaint.

An appeal against an attachment of earnings order is made to a divisional court of the Family Division of the High Court.

It may be desirable before taking any enforcement proceedings to obtain an order for oral examination of the debtor. The purpose of the examination is to establish what debts are owing to him or her and what other property he or she has. An application can then be made in the divorce county court nearest to the place where the debtor resides or works. If the debtor fails to appear for the appointment notice of a further appointment will be given and served with five clear days' notice of the rehearing date. There will be a risk of commitment to prison if the debtor again fails to appear. The order made provides for payment to be made to the court. The debtor may be ordered to produce books and documents to verify his or her evidence.

Another method of obtaining regular payments is by a matrimonial judgment summons. This is made in the county court and does not involve the debtor's employers. The procedure is set out in the *Family Proceedings Rules* 1991 (see Rayden on divorce 17th edition for complete text). An order made for lump sums, periodical payments and maintenance for children can be enforced in this way, but not an order for costs. The procedure involves filing a request in form M16 with an affidavit verifying the money due under the order. The court summons is in form M17 and has to be personally served on the debtor not less than five clear days before the hearing, for which the debtor must be given travel expenses. The purpose of the summons is to ensure that the debtor can be examined on oath as to his or her means. An order can be made without the debtor's attendance.

If the order to be enforced in this way is a maintenance order for children, the parent with whom they live has to apply on their behalf as their next friend and the solicitor has to provide a certificate of his or her fitness to act. One summons is issued in respect of each child.

The judge may make a new order, which will be for the payment of the amount due and the costs of the summons by instalments. If there is default a further summons can be issued with a view to commitment to prison for failure to attend.

Where an order for commitment to prison is made notice is sent to the debtor, and a debtor who does not respond may be arrested. A sentence of up to six weeks can be imposed.

Recovery of the entire amount of the debt is by any of the three following methods.

A warrant of execution is applied for in a county court where the amount owing is up to £5,000; or, if it is more than £5,000, in the High Court, and proceedings must be by way of a writ of *fi.fa.* (the full term is *fieri facias*): a summons supported by an affidavit setting out grounds has to be served four clear days before the date on which the order is to be made. If an order is made execution is levied by court bailiffs against the debtor's goods.

Under the Charging Orders Act 1979, where a large lump sum is payable or amounts of periodical payments have accumulated an application can be made to the district judge which does not have to be served on the debtor (this is called an ex-parte application) with a supporting affidavit to the district judge. The purpose of the application is to impose a charge on the debtor's land pursuant to the Act. If for example the debtor owns a house which is mortgaged, the debt will be a charge which can be paid to the creditor after the first debt has been paid. It will only be made if it is likely that there will be enough equity in the property. The mortgagees of the property must be identified in the affidavit. If when the order is made the payment is not made by the debtor a sale can be forced by the creditor and the net proceeds will be paid to the court.

Applications for garnishee orders are made by the same method. An application is made supported by an affidavit as to the amount unpaid under the order; and interest is claimed from the date of default in the payment. The purpose of the application is to seize accounts or funds due to the debtor by a third party, for example bank accounts but not employers' salary accounts. The summons issued is returnable in three weeks because the garnishee, that is the bank or the contractor, must be served at least 15 days before the hearing of the application so that he or she can appear at it. The costs of the garnishee will be included in the order if it is made, and the order is for the garnishee to make payments direct to the creditor.

Arrears of child maintenance under assessments are pursued by the Child Support Agency's administrative officers, who can make administrative orders known as 'deduction of earnings orders'. No court is involved in the procedure. The obligations of the employer are similar to the rules relating to the normal deduction rate and protected earnings rate applied in attachment of earnings cases. The second method employed by the Agency is to obtain liability orders where deduction is inappropriate (for example where the debtor is unemployed). An application is made to the Magistrates' Court by a child support officer for a liability order and if it is not complied with, enforcement can be levied by a process called 'distress'. It is the same as execution: it involves seizure and sale of a debtor's goods to the extent of his debt; but whereas an application to the court has to be made for a warrant of execution the court is not involved in the process of distraint under the Child Support legislation. What happens is a purely administrative procedure. The agency employs private bailiffs. They seize goods to the amount of the value owing on the assessments. Any irregularities which result in special damage may be claimed in trespass proceedings but the child support officers are not committing trespass by entering the premises in order to distrain goods.

The Agency can also use garnishee proceedings or apply for a charging order (Section 36 Child Support Act 1991). If either distress or a charging order or a garnishee order results in part of the maintenance being unpaid, an application can be made for the debtor's committal to prison but this has to be made to a court. This court is obliged to enquire into the person's means and state whether there has been wilful refusal or neglect in failing to comply with the assessment (Child Support Act 1991 Section 40). The period of imprisonment imposed can be up to six weeks. No legal aid is available for a debtor in relation to a child maintenance assessment.

Notice of severance of joint tenancy

TO: **James Smith**

OF: **1 Acacia Avenue, Tottingdean, Hamptonshire**

TAKE NOTICE that the joint tenancy which has hitherto subsisted between yourself and Mavis Smith with regard to the property, details of which appear in the Schedule hereto, is hereby severed and that henceforth the property is to be held as tenants in common.

THE SCHEDULE

ALL THAT land situate and known as 1 Acacia Avenue, Tottingdean, Hampstonshire and registered at HM Land Registry with title absolute under title number HS964321.

Dated this 6th day of November 1995

Solicitors for the above named Mavis Smith

I acknowledge receipt of the notice of severance of joint tenancy of which this is a true copy.

Signed . . . .
James Smith

Dated:

Evans and Evans (practice note) Family Division (26 January 1990)

Booth J. This is a wife's application for ancillary relief following upon a divorce. She seeks for herself a clean financial break from the husband and for the two minor children of the family who live with her she seeks periodical payments. The case has caused me anxiety because of the enormity of the costs which have been incurred in comparison with the assets which are available to meet the needs of the parties. On the husband's side the costs amount in all to £35,000 and on the wife's side they are estimated at £25,000. The available assets consist broadly of two properties both subject to mortgages which are the homes of the respective parties and the husband's shareholding in a small company which provides his livelihood and that of the children and which will not be sold in the foreseeable future. The wife is legally aided and has no independent means. It will thus be seen that the costs are out of all proportion to the assets.

This is by no means an isolated case in this respect. The situation recurs again and again when the court finds itself unable to make appropriate provision for the parties and their children because of their liability for legal costs and it is a matter of the gravest concern to all judges. With the concurrence of the President of the Family Division I shall commence my judgment with some general guidelines to be followed by the practitioner in the preparation of a substantial ancillary relief case.

1. Affidavit evidence should be confined to relevant facts and should not be prolix or diffuse. Each party should normally file one substantive affidavit dealing with the matters to which the court should have record under Section 25 of the Matrimonial Causes Act 1973, as substituted by Section 3 of the Matrimonial

and Family Proceedings Act 1984, and matters which are material to the application. If any further affidavit is necessary it should be confined to such matters as answering any serious allegation made by the other party, dealing with any serious issue raised or setting out any material change of circumstances.

2. Inquiries made under rule 77 (now FPR, r.2.63) of the Matrimonial Causes Rules 1977 should, as far as possible, be contained in one comprehensive questionnaire and should not be made piecemeal at different times.

3. Wherever possible valuations of properties should be obtained from a valuer instructed by both parties. Where each party instructs a valuer then reports should be exchanged and the valuers should meet in an attempt to resolve any differences between them or otherwise to narrow the issues.

4. While it may be necessary to obtain a broad assessment of the value of a shareholding in a private company it is inappropriate to undertake an expensive and meaningless exercise to achieve a precise valuation of a private company which will not be sold: see *P* v. *P* 1989 2 FLR 241.

5. All professional witnesses should be careful to avoid a partisan approach and should maintain proper professional standards.

6. Care should be taken in deciding what evidence, other than professional evidence, should be adduced and emotive issues which are not material to the case should be avoided. Where affidavit evidence is filed the deponents must be available for cross-examination on notice from the other side.

7. Solicitors on both sides should together prepare bundles of documents for use at the hearing and should reach agreement as to what should be included and what excluded: duplication of documents should always be avoided.

8. A chronology of material facts should be agreed and made available to the court.

9. In a substantial case it may be desirable to have a pre-trial review to explore the possibility of settlement and to define the issues and to ensure readiness for hearing if a settlement cannot be reached.

10. Solicitors and Counsel should keep their clients informed of the cost at all stages of the proceedings and, where appropriate, should ensure that they understand the implications of the legal aid charge: the court will require an estimate of the approximate amount of the costs on each side before it can make a lump sum

award: see Practice Direction (Divorce Registry: Lump Sum Award) 1982 1 WLR 1082.

11. The desirability of reaching a settlement should be borne in mind throughout the proceedings. While it is necessary for the legal advisers to have sufficient knowledge of the financial situation of both parties before advising their client on a proposed settlement, the necessity to make further inquiries must always be balanced by a consideration of what they are realistically likely to achieve and the increased costs which are likely to be incurred by making them.

Appendix 3

List of divorce courts in England and Wales*

Aberystwyth County Court
Eddleston House
Queens Road
Aberystwyth
Dyfed SY23 2HP
Tel: 01970 617597
Fax: 01970 625985

Accrington County Court
1st Floor
Bradshawgate House
1 Oak Street
Accrington
Lancashire BB5 1EQ
Tel: 01254 237490
Fax: 01254 393869

Aldershot and Farnham
County Court
78–82 Victoria Road
Aldershot
Hampshire GU11 1SS
Tel: 01252 21639
Fax: 01252 345705

Andover Court Court
2nd Floor
Chantry House
Chantry Way
Andover
Hampshire SP10 1NB
Tel: 01264 366622
Fax: 01264 338983

Barnet County Court
St Mary's Court
Regents Park Road
Finchley Central
London N3 1BQ
Tel: 0181 343 4272
Fax: 0181 343 1324

Barnsley County Court
12 Regent Street
Barnsley
South Yorkshire S70 2EW
Tel: 01226 203471
Fax: 01226 779126

*Reproduced by kind permission of the Solicitors Family Law Association from their *Divorce Court Guide 1994 (Family Law)*

Barrow-in-Furness County
Court
Government Buildings
Michaelson Road
Barrow-in-Furness
Cumbria LA14 2EX
Tel: 01229 820046/827150
Fax: 01229 430039

Basingstoke County Court
3rd Floor
Grosvenor House
Basing View
Basingstoke
Hampshire RG21 2HG
Tel: 01256 22754
Fax: 01256 57131

Bath County Court
3rd & 4th Floors
Cambridge House
Henry Street
Bath
Avon BA1 1DJ
Tel: 01225 310282
Fax: 01225 480915

Bedford County Court
29 Goldington Road
Bedford
Bedfordshire MK40 3NN
Tel: 01234 359322
Fax: 01234 327431

Birkenhead County Court
76 Hamilton Street
Birkenhead
Merseyside L41 3EN
Tel: 0151 647 8826/7
Fax: 0151 647 3501

Birmingham County Court
2 Newton Street
Birmingham
West Midlands B4 7LU
Tel: 0121 627 1700
Fax: 0121 212 1328

Bishop Auckland County
Court
Saddler House
Saddler Street
Bishop Auckland
Durham DL14 7HF
Tel: 01388 602423

Blackburn County Court
64 Victoria Street
Blackburn
Lancashire BB1 6DJ
Tel: 01254 680640
Fax: 01254 692712

Blackpool County Court
The Law Courts
Chapel Street
Blackpool
Lancashire FY1 5RJ
Tel: 01253 293178
Fax: 01253 295253

Blackwood County Court
Blackwood Road
Blackwood
Gwent NP2 2XB
Tel: 01495 223197
Fax: 01495 220289

Bodmin County Court
Cockswell House
Market Street
Bodmin
Cornwall PL31 2HJ
Tel: 01208 74224
Fax: 01208 77255

Bolton County Court
The Law Courts
Blackhorse Street
Bolton
Lancashire BL1 1SU
Tel: 01204 392881
Fax: 01204 363204

Boston County Court
Crown Building
Lincoln Lane
Boston
Lincolnshire PE21 8SG
Tel: 01205 366080
Fax: 01205 311692

Bournemouth County Court
The Law Courts (Old
  Buildings)
Stafford Road
Bournemouth
Dorset BH1 1PN
Tel: 01202 553701
Fax: 01202 290819

Bow County Court
96 Romford Road
Stratford
London E15 4EG
Tel: 0181 555 3421
Fax: 0181 503 1152

Bradford County Court
Bradford Law Courts
Exchange Square
Drake Street
Bradford
West Yorkshire BD1 1JA
Tel: 01274 840274
Fax: 01274 840275

Brentford County Court
Alexandra Road
Brentford
Middlesex TW8 OJJ
Tel: 0181 560 3424
Fax: 0181 568 2401

Bridgend County Court
Crown Buildings
Angel Street
Bridgend
Mid Glamorgan CF31 4AS
Tel: 01656 768881
Fax: 01656 647124

Brighton County Court
William Street
Brighton
East Sussex BN2 2LG
Tel: 01273 674421
Fax: 01273 602138

Bristol County Court
Greyfriars
Lewins Mead
Bristol
Avon BS1 2NR
Tel: 01179 294414
Fax: 01179 250912

Bromley County Court
The Court House
College Road
Bromley
Kent BR1 3PX
Tel: 0181 464 9727
Fax: 0181 313 9624

Burnley County Court
Burnley Combined Court
  Centre
The Law Courts
Hammerton Street
Burnley
Lancashire BB1 1XD
Tel: 01282 416889
Fax: 01282 414911

Burton-upon-Trent County
  Court
165 Station Street
Burton-upon-Trent
Staffordshire
DE14 1BP
Tel: 01283 568241
Fax: 01283 517245

Bury County Court
Tenterden Street
Bury
Lancashire BL9 0HJ
Tel: 0161 764 1344
Fax: 0161 763 4995

Bury St Edmunds County
  Court
Triton House
Entrance B
St Andrews Street North
Bury St Edmunds
Suffolk IP33 1TR
Tel: 01284 753254
Fax: 01284 702687

Caernarfon County Court
Government Buildings
North Penralt
Caernarfon
Gwynedd LL55 1PR
Tel: 01286 678911
Fax: 01286 678965

Camborne and Redruth
  County Court
The Josiah Thomas Memorial
Hall
Fore Street
Camborne
Cornwall TR14 8AY
Tel: 01209 715585
Fax: 01209 715075

Cambridge County Court
Three Crowns House
72/80 Hills Road
Cambridge
Cambridgeshire CB2 1LA
Tel: 01223 354416
Fax: 01223 324775

Canterbury County Court
Riding Gate House
37 Old Dover Road
Canterbury
Kent CT1 3JD
Tel: 01227 462383
Fax: 01227 766752

Cardiff County Court
PO Box 64
Government Buildings
Westgate Street
Cardiff
South Glamorgan CF1 1NR
Tel: 01222 395631
Fax: 01222 382677

Carmarthen County Court
The Old Vicarage
Picton Terrace
Carmarthen
Dyfed SA31 1BJ
Tel: 01267 236598
Fax: 01267 221844

Chelmsford County Court
London House
New London Road
Chelmsford
Essex CM2 0QR
Tel: 01245
264670/281386/350718
Fax: 01245 496216

Chester County Court
First Floor
Centurion House
77 Northgate Street
Chester
Cheshire CH1 2HQ
Tel: 01244 312245
Fax: 01244 315635

Chesterfield County Court
49 Church Way
Chesterfield
Derbyshire S40 1SG
Tel: 01246 232191/278963
Fax: 01246 557297

Chichester County Court
Chichester Combined Court
  Centre
The Court House
Southgate
Chichester
West Sussex PO19 1SX
Tel: 01243 786151
Fax: 01243 533756

Chippenham County Court
Kilvert House
Greenways Park
Bellinger Close
Chippenham
Wiltshire SN15 1BJ
Tel: 01249 655111
Fax: 01249 446389

Chorley County Court
59 St Thomas's Road
Chorley
Lancashire PR7 1JE
Tel: 01257 262778
Fax: 01257 232843

Colchester County Court
Falkland House
25 Southway
Colchester
Essex CO3 3EG
Tel: 01206 572743
Fax: 01206 369610

Coventry County Court
Coventry Combined Court
  Centre
140 Much Park Street
Coventry
West Midlands CV1 2SN
Tel: 01203 536166
Fax: 01203 520443

Crewe County Court
The Law Courts
Civic Centre
Crewe
Cheshire CW1 2DP
Tel: 01270 212255
Fax: 01270 216344

Darlington County Court
4 Coniscliffe Road
Darlington
Durham DL3 7RL
Tel: 01325 463224
Fax: 01325 362829

Derby County Court
Derby Combined Court Centre
The Morledge
Derbyshire DE1 2XE
Tel: 01332 622600
Fax: 01332 622543

Dewsbury County Court
County Court House
Eightlands Road
Dewsbury
West Yorkshire WF13 2PE
Tel: 01924 466135
Fax: 01924 456419

Doncaster County Court
74 Waterdale
Doncaster
South Yorkshire DN1 3BT
Tel: 01302 365400
Fax: 01302 768090

Dudley County Court
61 The Broadway
Dudley
West Midlands DY1 3EF
Tel: 01384 236321
Fax: 01384 257579

Edmonton County Court
Court House
59 Fore Street
Upper Edmonton
London N18 2NT
Tel: 0181 807 1666
Fax: 0181 803 0564

Epsom County Court
The Parade
Epsom
Surrey KT18 5DN
Tel: 01372 721802
Fax: 01372 726588

Exeter County Court
The Castle
Exeter
Devon EX4 3DS
Tel: 01392 210655
Fax: 01392 433546

Gateshead County Court
5th Floor
Chad House
Tynegate Precinct
Gateshead
Tyne and Wear NE8 3HZ
Tel: 0191 477 2445
Fax: 0191 478 8562

Gloucester County Court
Barton House
121–127 Eastgate Street
Gloucester
Gloucestershire GL1 1QL
Tel: 01452 529351
Fax: 01452 386309

Great Grimsby County Court
Great Grimsby Combined
  Court Centre
Town Hall Square
Grimsby
Humberside DN31 1HX
Tel: 01472 345816
Fax: 01472 241288

Guildford County Court
The Law Courts
Mary Road
Guildford
Surrey GU1 4PS
Tel: 01483 34991
Fax: 01483 300031

Halifax County Court
The Courthouse
Prescott Street
Halifax
West Yorkshire HX1 2JJ
Tel: 01422 352924/355910
Fax: 01422 360132

Harlow County Court
Gate House
The High
Harlow
Essex CM20 1UW
Tel: 01279 442391
Fax: 01279 451110

Harrogate County Court
12a North Park Road
Harrogate
North Yorkshire HG1 5PY
Tel: 01423
503921/564837/524520
Fax: 01423 528679

Hartlepool County Court
 Law Courts
Victoria Road
Hartlepool
Cleveland TS24 8BS
Tel: 01429 268198
Fax: 01429 862550

Hastings County Court
The Law Courts
Bohemia Road
Hastings
East Sussex TN34 1QX
Tel: 01424 435128
Fax: 01424 421585

Haverfordwest County Court
Crown Buildings
Cherry Grove
Haverfordwest
Dyfed SA61 2NN
Tel: 01437 765741/2
Fax: 01437 769222

Hertford County Court
Sovereign House
Hale Road
Hertford
Hertfordshire SG13 8DY
Tel: 01992 503594
Fax: 01992 501274

Hitchin County Court
Park House
1–12 Old Park Road
Hitchin
Hertfordshire SG5 1LX
Tel: 01462 432418/450011
Fax: 01462 432161

Horsham County Court
The Law Courts
Hurst Road
Horsham
West Sussex RH12 2GU
Tel: 01403 252474
Fax: 01403 258844

Ilford County Court
Buckingham Road
Ilford
Essex IG1 1BR
Tel: 0181 478 1132/4
Fax: 0181 553 2824

Ipswich County Court
8 Arcade Street
Ipswich
Suffolk IP1 1EJ
Tel: 01473 214256
Fax: 01473 251797

Keighley County Court
Yorkshire Bank Chambers
North Street
Keighley
West Yorkshire BD21 3SH
Tel: 01535 602803
Fax: 01535 610549

King's Lynn County Court
The Court House
London Road
King's Lynn
Norfolk PE30 5PU
Tel: 01553 772067
Fax: 01553 769824

Kingston upon Hull County
  Court
Combined Court Centre
Lowgate
Kingston upon Hull
Humberside HU1 2EZ
Tel: 01482 586161
Fax: 01482 588527

Kingston upon Thames County
Court
St James Road
Kingston upon Thames
Surrey KT1 2AD
Tel: 0181 546 8843
Fax: 0181 547 1426

Leeds County Court
The Courthouse
1 Oxford Row
Leeds
West Yorkshire LS1 3BG
Tel: 0113 2830040
Fax: 0113 2448507

Leicester County Court
Lower Hill Street
Leicester
Leicestershire LE1 3SJ
Tel: 0116 2653400
Fax: 0116 2653450

Leigh County Court
22 Walmesley Road
Leigh
Lancashire WN7 1YE
Tel: 01942 673639
Fax: 01942 681216

Lincoln Combined Court
360 High Street
Lincoln
Lincolnshire LN5 7RL
Tel: 01522 521500
Fax: 01522 511150

Liverpool County Court
Queen Elizabeth II Law
  Courts
Derby Square
Liverpool
Merseyside L2 1XA
Tel: 0151 473 7373
Fax: 0151 227 2806

Llanelli County Court
2nd Floor
Court Buildings
Town Hall Square
Llanelli
Dyfed SA15 3AL
Tel: 01554 757171
Fax: 01554 758079

Llangefni County Court
County Court Buildings
Glanhwfa Road
Llangefni
Gwynedd LL77 7EN
Tel: 01248 750225
Fax: 01248 750778

Lowestoft County Court
28 Gordon Road
Lowestoft
Suffolk NR32 1NL
Tel: 01502 573701/586047
Fax: 01502 569319

Luton County Court
2nd Floor
Cresta House
Alma Street
Luton
Bedfordshire LU1 2PU
Tel: 01582 35671
Fax: 01582 24752

Maidstone County Court
The Law Courts
Barker Road
Maidstone
Kent ME16 8EQ
Tel: 01622 754966
Fax: 01622 687349

Manchester County Court
Courts of Justice
Crown Square
Manchester M60 9DJ
Tel: 0161 954 1800
Fax: 0161 839 2756

Mansfield County Court
Clerkson House
St Peters Way
Mansfield
Nottinghamshire NG18 1BQ
Tel: 01623 656406
Fax: 01623 26561

Medway County Court
Anchorage House
47–67 High Street
Chatham
Kent ME4 4DW
Tel: 01634 402881
Fax: 01634 811332

Merthyr Tydfil County Court
The Law Courts
Glebeland Place
Merthyr Tydfil
Mid Glamorgan CF47 8BH
Tel: 01685 721322
Fax: 01685 359727

Milton Keynes County Court
351 Silbury Boulevard
Witan Gate East
Central Milton Keynes
Buckinghamshire MK9 2DT
Tel: 01908 668855
Fax: 01908 230063

Neath and Port Talbot County
  Court
County Court Office
Forster Road
Neath
West Glamorgan SA11 3BN
Tel: 01639 642267
Fax: 01639 633505

Nelson County Court
Phoenix Chambers
9–13 Holme Street
Nelson
Lancashire BB9 9SU
Tel: 01282 601177
Fax: 01282 619557

Newcastle upon Tyne County
  Court
The Law Courts
Quayside
Newcastle upon Tyne
Tyne and Wear NE1 3LA
Tel: 0191 201 2000
Fax: 0191 201 2001

Newport (Gwent) County
  Court
Olympia House
3rd Floor
Upper Dock Street
Newport
Gwent NP9 1PQ
Tel: 01633 255267
Fax: 01633 263820

Newport (IOW) County Court
  Combined Court Centre
130/132 High Street
Newport
Isle of Wight PO30 1TP
Tel: 01983 526821
Fax: 01983 821039

North Shields County Court
Northumbria House
Norfolk Street
North Shields
Tyne and Wear NE30 1EX
Tel: 0191 257 5866
Fax: 0191 296 4268

Northampton Combined Court
85–87 Lady's Lane
Northampton NN1 3HR
Tel: 01604 250131
Fax: 01604 31853

Norwich Combined Court
The Law Courts
Bishopgate
Norwich
Norfolk NR3 1UR
Tel: 01603 761776
Fax: 01603 760863

Nottingham County Court
Nottingham Combined Court
  Centre
60 Canal Street
Nottingham
Nottinghamshire NG1 7EJ
Tel: 0115 9793500
Fax: 0115 9793588

Oldham County Court
Church Lane
Oldham
Lancashire OL1 3AR
Tel: 0161 620 0425
Fax: 0161 620 0605

Oxford County Court
Oxford Combined County
  Court Centre
St Aldates
Oxford
Oxfordshire OX1 1TL
Tel: 01865 264200
Fax: 01865 790773

Penrith County Court
The Court House
Lowther Terrace
Penrith
Cumbria CA11 7QL
Tel: 01768 62535
Fax: 01768 899700

Peterborough Combined
  County Court
Crown Buildings
Rivergate
Peterborough
Cambridgeshire PE1 1FJ
Tel: 01733 349161
Fax 01733 557348

Plymouth County Court
Combined Court Centre
The Law Courts
Armada Way
Plymouth
Devon PL1 2ER
Tel: 01752 674808
Fax: 01752 661447

Pontypridd County Court
The Court House
Courthouse Street
Pontypridd
Mid Glamorgan CF37 1JW
Tel: 01443 402471
Fax: 01443 480305

Portsmouth County Court
Courts of Justice
Winston Churchill Avenue
Portsmouth
Hampshire PO1 2EB
Tel: 01705 822281
Fax: 01705 826385

Preston County Court
Robert House
2 Starkie Street
Preston
Lancashire PR1 3HB
Tel: 01772 252024/250220
Fax: 01772 882554

Rawtenstall County Court
1 Grance Street
Rawtenstall
Rossendale
Lancashire BB4 7RT
Tel: 01706 214614
Fax: 01706 219814

Reading County Court
160–163 Friar Street
Reading
Berkshire RG1 1HB
Tel: 01734 599833
Fax: 01734 391892

Reigate County Court
Hatchlands Road
Redhill
Surrey RH1 6BL
Tel: 01737 763637
Fax: 01737 766917

Rhyl County Court
64 Brighton Road
Rhyl
Clwyd LL18 3HR
Tel: 01745 330216
Fax: 01745 336726

Romford County Court
2a Oaklands Avenue
Romford
Essex RM1 4DP
Tel: 01708 750677
Fax: 01708 756653

Rotherham County Court
Portland House
Mansfield Road
Rotherham
South Yorkshire S60 2BX
Tel: 01709 365544/364786
Fax: 01709 838044

Runcorn County Court
The Law Courts
Shopping City
Runcorn
Cheshire WA7 2HA
Tel: 01928 716533
Fax: 01928 701692

St Helens County Court
1st Floor
Rexmore House
Cotham Street
St Helens
Merseyside WA10 1SE
Tel: 01744 27544
Fax: 01744 20484

Salford County Court
Prince William House
Peel Cross Road
Salford M5 2RR
Tel: 0161 834 9474/1614
Fax: 0161 839 2489

Scarborough County Court
9 Northway
Scarborough
North Yorkshire YO11 2EH
Tel: 01723 366361
Fax: 01723 501992

Scunthorpe County Court
Crown Buildings
Comforts Avenue
Scunthorpe
South Humberside DN15 6PR
Tel: 01724 855395/871345
Fax: 01724 271669

Sheffield Combined Court
  Centre
The Law Courts
50 West Bar
Sheffield
South Yorkshire S3 8PH
Tel: 0114 2812400
Fax: 0114 2812425

Shrewsbury County Court
3rd Floor
Mardol House
Market Hall Buildings
Shoplatch
Shrewsbury
Shropshire
Tel: 01743 232650
Fax: 01743 244479

Skipton County Court
The Court House
Otley Street
Skipton
North Yorkshire BD23 1EH
Tel: 01756 793315
Fax: 01756 799989

Slough County Court
The Law Courts
Windsor Road
Slough
Berkshire SL1 2HE
Tel: 01753 522307
Fax: 01753 575990

South Shields County Court
25–26 Market Place
South Shields
Tyne and Wear NE33 1AG
Tel: 0191 456 3343
Fax: 0191 427 9503

Southampton County Court
The Courts of Justice
London Road
Southampton
Hampshire SO9 5AF
Tel: 01703 228586
Fax: 01703 339772

Southend County Court
Tylers House
Tylers Avenue
Southend on Sea
Essex SS1 2AW
Tel: 01702 601991
Fax: 01702 603090

Southport County Court
Dukes House
34 Hoghton Street
Southport
Merseyside PR9 0PU
Tel: 01704 531541
Fax: 01704 542487

Stafford County Court
Stafford Combined Court
  Centre
Victoria Square
Stafford
Staffordshire ST16 2QQ
Tel: 01785 255217
Fax: 01785 213250

Staines County Court
The Law Courts
Knowle Green
Staines
Middlesex TW18 1XH
Tel: 01784 459175
Fax: 01784 460176

Stockport County Court
5th Floor
Heron House
Wellington Street
Stockport
Cheshire SK1 3DJ
Tel: 0161 480 7911/6443
Fax: 0161 476 3129

Stockton-on-Tees County
  Court
4 Bridge Road
Stockton-on-Tees
Cleveland TS18 3BS
Tel: 01642 612831
Fax: 01642 615994

Stoke-on-Trent County Court
Bethesda Street
Hanley
Stoke-on-Trent
Staffordshire ST1 3BP
Tel: 01782 215076
Fax: 01782 213492

Sunderland County Court
44 John Street
Sunderland
Tyne and Wear SR1 1RB
Tel: 0191 567 3691
Fax: 0191 514 3028

Swansea County Court
Government Buildings
10 St Mary's Square
Swansea
West Glamorgan SA1 3LL
Tel: 01792 472244
Fax: 01792 463444

Swindon County Court
The Law Courts
Islington Street
Swindon
Wiltshire SN1 2HG
Tel: 01793 614848
Fax: 01793 618076

Tameside County Court
Scotland Street
Aston-under-Lyne
Lancashire OL6 6SS
Tel: 0161 339 1711
Fax: 0161 339 1645

Taunton County Court
Shire Hall
Taunton
Somerset TA1 4EU
Tel: 01823 335972
Fax: 01823 322116

Teeside County Court
Teeside Combined Court
  Centre
Russell Street
Middlesbrough
Cleveland TS1 2AE
Tel: 01642 340000
Fax: 01642 340002

Telford County Court
Telford Square
Malinsgate Town Centre
Telford
Shropshire TF3 4JP
Tel: 01952 291045
Fax: 01952 291601

Torquay County Court
Castle Chambers
Union Street
Torquay
Devon TQ1 4BS
Tel: 01803 294084
Fax: 01803 290470

Trowbridge County Court
Ground Floor
Clarks Mill
Stallard Street
Trowbridge
Wiltshire BA14 8DB
Tel: 01225 752101
Fax: 01225 776638

Tunbridge Wells County Court
Merevale House
42–46 London Road
Tunbridge Wells
Kent TN1 1DN
Tel: 01892 515515
Fax: 01892 513676

Uxbridge County Court
114 High Street
Uxbridge
Middlesex
Tel: 01895 230441
Fax: 01895 232261

Wakefield County Court
The Court House
127 Kirkgate
Wakefield
West Yorkshire WF1 1JW
Tel: 01924 370268
Fax: 01924 200818

Walsall County Court
Bridge House
Bridge Street
Walsall
West Midlands WS1 1JQ
Tel: 01922 432250
Fax: 01922 432316

Wandsworth County Court
76–78 Richmond Road
Putney
London SW15 2SU
Tel: 0181 870 2212
Fax: 0181 877 9854

Watford County Court
Casslobury House
11–19 Station Road
Watford
Hertfordshire WD1 1EZ
Tel: 01923 249666
Fax: 01923 251317

West Bromwich County Court
Second Floor
Spencer House
355–357 High Street
West Bromwich
West Midlands B70 8RF
Tel: 0121 500 5101
Fax: 0121 580 0115

Weston-super-Mare County
Court
Second Floor
Regent House
High Street
Weston-super-Mare
Avon BS23 1JF
Tel: 01934 626967
Fax: 01934 643028

Weymouth County Court
2nd Floor
Westwey House
Westwey Road
Weymouth
Dorset DT4 8TE
Tel: 01305 778684
Fax: 01305 788293

Whitehaven County Court
Old Town Hall
Duke Street
Whitehaven
Cumbria CA28 7NV
Tel: 01946 67788
Fax: 01946 691219

Wigan County Court
The Court House
Crawford Street
Wigan
Lancashire WN1 1NG
Tel: 01942 246481
Fax: 01942 829164

Winchester County Court
Winchester Combined Court
  Centre
The Law Courts
Winchester
Hampshire SO23 9EL
Tel: 01962 841212
Fax: 01962 853821

Wolverhampton County Court
Wolverhampton Combined
  Court Centre
Pipers Row
Wolverhampton
West Midlands WV61 3LQ
Tel: 01902 481000
Fax: 01902 21526

Worcester County Court
Sandwell House
48 Foregate Street
Worcester
Hereford and Worcester
WR1 1EQ
Tel: 01905 730800
Fax: 01905 723064

Worthing County Court
The Law Courts
Christchurch Road
Worthing
West Sussex BN11 1JD
Tel: 01903 206721
Fax: 01903 23559

Wrexham County Court
2nd Floor
31 Chester Street
Wrexham
Clwyd LL13 8XN
Tel: 01978 351738
Fax: 01978 290677

Yeovil County Court
20 Kingston
Yeovil
Somerset BA20 2QD
Tel: 01935 74133
Fax: 01935 410004

York County Court
Aldwark House
Aldwark
off Goodramgate
York
North Yorkshire YO1 2BX
Tel: 01904 629935
Fax: 01904 679963

Appendix 4

Pensions and divorce*

One of the most intractable problems in divorce proceedings is valuing the pension rights and expectations of the parties.

Reform of the law through a system of pension splitting on divorce has now been recommended by the Pensions Management Institute (PMI) in its 1993 report *Pensions and Divorce*, and by the pension law review committee chaired by Professor Goode in its subsequent report *Pension Law Reform*, produced in September 1993.

The PMI report suggested that the best way to value pensions was by using transfer values. This is backed up by the decision in *H* v. *H* (Financial Provision: Capital Allowance) (1993) 2 FLR 335, that reference should be made to pension rights which accrued during the marriage.

In order to assist practitioners in the meantime, the family law committee thought it might be useful to have to hand a form of letter of instruction to an actuary to value the pension interests of the parties together with a questionnaire for use under FPR 2.63 (as amended).

An actuary should only be instructed where the use of transfer values is not thought to be appropriate. In cases where an expert accountant has already been instructed, consideration should be given to instructing him or her to value any pension rights.

The first draft of these documents has appeared in the *Gazette* (see *Gazette*, 13 January 1993, p. 34). The draft set out below has been amended in the light of comments received on that first draft. These documents do not purport to be conclusive or a standard,

* Reprinted by permission of the Law Society, from *The Law Society's Gazette*, July, 6 (1994).

and obviously may be amended to suit individual circumstances. They are only appropriate for use under English law and relate only to occupational pension schemes.

When reading them, reference should therefore be made to the recent case of *Brooks* v. *Brooks* (1994) *The Times*, 27 May.

LETTER OF INSTRUCTION TO ACTUARY TO VALUE OCCUPATIONAL PENSION RIGHTS

Our Ref:

Dear Sirs

1. We act for the person named below in divorce proceeding whose spouse is a member of the pension arrangements mentioned below.
2. We would be grateful for your opinion as to the value of the following losses which would be suffered by our client following a decree absolute of divorce as at (xx):

   loss of survivor's pension;
   loss of interest in the spouse's pension;
   loss of interest in death benefits.

3. We enclose:

   copy of the explanatory booklet relating to the scheme;
   information provided by the spouse's solicitors;
   copy of a questionnaire served on the spouse's solicitors and the answers;
   copy of the latest annual benefit statement of the spouse.

4. We set out below some information which you will require.

   name of client in full: (m/f) and date of birth;
   name of spouse in full: (m/f) and date of birth;
   name of occupational pension scheme;
   date of marriage;
   names of children and date of birth;
   spouse's salary;
   spouse's pensionable salary;
   spouse's date of commencement of employment;
   spouse's date of joining scheme (if different);
   spouse's unfunded pension arrangements.

5. Please let us know if you require any further information, and let us have an estimate of your charges before undertaking your valuation.

Yours faithfully

Notes on completing this letter

General notes

You will need a separate letter for each occupational pension scheme involved as the spouse may have pension arrangements with a series of occupational schemes. This letter is not designed to cater for personal pension contracts.

You can find a consulting actuary by writing to either the Association of Consulting Actuaries or the Institute of Actuaries.

In the case of insured pension arrangements (and for that matter all other pension arrangements) failure to disclose the required information in a reasonable time can be resolved either by use of the Occupational Pension Schemes (Disclosure of Information) Regulations 1986 (SI 86/1046) as amended by SI 86/1717 or, where this is not appropriate, by serving a notice on the pensions manager, or insurance company under Family Proceedings Rules 1991 (as amended) r.2.62(7) for them to attend on a 'production appointment'.

This document is not appropriate for state pension benefits. You can obtain information about state benefits by sending form BR19 to the Department of Social Security, in Newcastle upon Tyne.

All pension schemes now have to register with the Registry of Occupational and Personal Pensions. Form PR4 can be used by anyone entitled to benefit from a pension scheme to trace information about it.

Footnotes

1. Please tick as appropriate – in most cases all this information will be required. The date to be given will usually be the date of the separation, although in some cases it may be appropriate to ask for the rights to be valued at a future date such as the normal retirement date; for instance where retirement is imminent.

    Advice on the method of valuation from the actuary should

be sought, although use of the cash equivalent approach (transfer values) may well be appropriate.
2. Please tick as appropriate.
3. See questionnaire under Family Proceedings Rules 1991 (as amended) r.2.63 (attached) approved by the family law committee.
4. You should ensure that this is the salary as used for pension purposes. It may differ from the member's basic pay or total earnings. If you are in doubt, set out the source of the information and the date at which the figure applies.
5. Details of any special terms includes pension rights or expectations, i.e. non-formalised or unfunded, which may be contained, for example, in the contract of employment or a side-letter, rather than in the pension scheme. Unfunded arrangements should be specifically mentioned, as should the risk of non-payment of such pensions.

THE PENSIONS QUESTIONNAIRE

Approved by the Law Society's family law committee; designed to comply with Family Proceedings Rules 1991 (as amended) r.2.63.

Please provide the following information relating to any pension rights or expectations in connection with the petitioner/respondent.

name of petitioner/respondent;
name of scheme(s);
copies of:

explanatory booklet;
benefit statement (not more than 12 months old);
notes of any material changes to this information;

details of transfers in from other schemes;
details of any special terms agreed with the employer not contained in information supplied above;
details of any additional voluntary contributions payable by the petitioner/respondent and of the nature of the benefits secured thereby;

Is the petitioner/respondent contracted out of the earnings related part of the state pension scheme by virtue of his or her membership of the scheme?

details of the trustees'/employer's policy regarding guaranteed/
discretionary increases including details of the last ten years'
pension increase practice. In the case of discretionary
increases, please supply a statement of practice;
normal retirement age;

statement from the trustees of each scheme (or other appropriate source) explaining and quantifying the projected benefits
on retirement both on the basis that contributions continue at
the present rate until retirement; and on the basis that no further contributions are made in relation to:

(a) lump sum payable in the event of death in service;
(b) the pension which the petitioner/respondent will receive
upon retirement at normal retirement age on the basis that
he or she does not elect to commute part of his/her pension
for a lump sum;
(d) the maximum lump sum which the petitioner/respondent
could receive in part commutation of his/her pension;
(e) the maximum pension payable from normal retirement date
in the event of such commutation;
(f) spouse's pension on death after retirement.

statement of current transfer value;
details of current medical conditions which might affect the
value of rights under the scheme.

Notes on completing this form

General notes

Most of this information can be legally required to be provided
to members of schemes under the Disclosure Regulations (Occupational Pension Schemes (Disclosure of Information) Regulations,
SI 86/1046 as amended by SI86/1717).

This questionnaire should not be sent as a matter of course; it is
appropriate only where, at the date of the hearing, there is a
reasonable expectation of significant pension losses, for instance,
loss of an enforceable widow's pension, where a return of premiums
on death is possible, where the parties have been married for some
time, where the respondent is in pensionable employment and
is nearing retirement, where the pension loss is more likely to be
significant either because of long pensionable service of the older

member, and where the salary is significant (or in the public sector where pensions may be significant in relation to earnings).

If the marriage is long-lasting, even lower paid spouses should be asked to complete the questionnaire; even a modest pension which cannot be settled by an adjustment of the other matrimonial property could be enough to hold up a decree nisi.

This applies particularly to pensions in the public sector (see e.g. *Parkes* v. *Parkes* (1971) 1 WLR 1481; *Le Marchant* v. *Le Marchant* (1977) 3 All ER p. 610). Reference should also be had to *Griffiths* v. *Dawson & Co.* (1993) 2 FLR p. 315, which stressed the importance of making an application under Section 10(2) of the Matrimonial Causes Act 1973 (as amended) where a petition is based on two or five years' separation.

Footnotes

1. A separate questionnaire should be simultaneously completed for each pension arrangement involved.
2. Details of any special terms includes pension rights or expectations (i.e. non-formalised or unfunded) which may be contained, for example, in the contracts of employment or a side-letter, rather than in the pension scheme. Unfunded arrangements should be specifically mentioned, as should the risk of non-payment of such pensions.
3. Normal retirement age is the age set down in the pension scheme; it should be the same as that in the contract of employment.
4. Under the disclosure regulations, pension scheme trustees may only be prepared to give figures under one of these bases. If this is the case, it is probably best to ask for a statement of projected benefits on the basis that no further contributions are made, particularly in light of the decision in *H* v. *H* (see above p. 169).
5. The current transfer value should be calculated on the basis of cash equivalents under the Transfer Regulations.

Actuaries are occasionally requested by solicitors to provide a model mandate authorising a pension scheme and/or insurance company to disclose information directly to them. A draft mandate for use in these circumstances is set out below.

To the trustees of the pension scheme

Dear Sirs

Valuation of pension

I,   residing at
hereby authorise and request you to release to consulting
actuaries,   any information they may require
regarding my pension benefits to enable a valuation thereof to
be prepared.

Please quote the reference at the head of this letter in any
correspondence.

Appendix 5*

A fictional case study of a divorce followed by the progress of an application for financial relief culminating in an agreed order**

The Petition of Alice Jane Roberts shows that:

1. On the 15 March 1972 the Petitioner Alice Jane Roberts (formerly Jones) was lawfully married to Ronald James Roberts at The Register Office Crowbury in the County of Dorset.

2. The Petitioner and the Respondent last lived together as husband and wife at 5 Woodside Meadstown Beamshire.

3. The Petitioner is domiciled in England and Wales. The Petitioner is a School teacher and resides at 5 Woodside Meadstown aforesaid and the Respondent is a Company Director and resides at Flat 9 Cherrytree Gardens Meadstown.

4. There are two children of the family now living namely David Roberts born on the 5 September 1978 and John Roberts born on the 11 November 1981.

5. No other child now living has been born to the Petitioner during the marriage.

6. There are or have been no previous proceedings in any court

---

* Copyright for the use of terms within this appendix has been granted. Crown Copyright is reproduced with the permission of the Controller of HMSO.
** Note this case is entirely fictional. Any resemblance to a real case is completely coincidental.

in England and Wales or elsewhere with reference to the marriage or to any children of the family or between the Petitioner and the Respondent with reference to any property of either or both of them.

7. There are or have been no applications under the Child Support Act 1991 for a maintenance assessment in respect of any child of the family.

8. There are no proceedings continuing in any country outside England and Wales which relate to the marriage or are capable of affecting its validity or subsistence.

9. The said marriage has broken down irretrievably.

10. The parties to the marriage have lived apart for a continuous period of at least two years immediately preceding the presentation of this petition and the Respondent consents to a decree being granted.

11. Due to irreconcilable differences the parties separated on 31 January 1992 and have lived apart since that date.

The Petitioner therefore prays:

(1) That the said marriage may be dissolved;

(2) That the Respondent Ronald James Roberts may be ordered to pay the costs of this suit;

(3) That she may be granted the following ancillary relief;

    (i) an order for maintenance pending suit)
    (ii) a periodical payments order   )
    (iii) a secured provision order   ) for herself
    (iv) a lump sum order   )
    (v) a property adjustment order   )

    (vi) a secured provision order   ) for the
    (vii) a lump sum order   ) children
    (viii) a property adjustment order   ) of the family

Grossfees & Co
Solicitors for the Petitioner

The name and address of the person who is to be served with this Petition is:

Respondent: Ronald James Roberts
               c/o Clements & Co.
               60 High Street
               Meadstown

The Petitioner's address for service is:

               c/o Grossfees & Co
               75 High Street
               Meadstown
               Beamshire

Dated 11 day of February 1994

IN THE PRINCIPAL REGISTRY*

No. 3554 of 1994

IN THE MATTER of the Petition of

ALICE JANE ROBERTS

DIVORCE PETITION

(Wife against Husband)

(2 years Separation – Consent)

---

* Note all backsheets appear at the back of documents in this appendix – as they
would on the solicitor's and court files.

| SPECIMEN |

No. 3554 of 94
IN THE PRINCIPAL REGISTRY
OF THE FAMILY DIVISION

BETWEEN	ALICE JANE ROBERTS	Petitioner
AND	RONALD JAMES ROBERTS	Respondent
AND		Co-Respondent

Notice of proceedings

A petition for divorce has been presented to this Court. A sealed copy of it and a copy of the petitioner's Statement of Arrangements for the child(ren) are delivered with this notice.

1. You must complete and detach the acknowledgment of service and send it so as to reach the court within 7 days after you receive this notice. Delay in returning the form may add to the costs.

2. If you intend to instruct a solicitor to act for you, you should at once give him all the documents which have been served on you, so that he may send the acknowledgment to the Court on your behalf. If you do not intend to instruct a solicitor, you should nevertheless give an address for service in the acknowledgement so that any documents affecting your interests which are sent to you will in fact reach you. Change of address should be notified to the Court.

Notes on questions in the acknowledgement of service

3. If you answer Yes to Question 4 you must within 28 days after you receive this notice, file in the Court office an answer to the petition together with a copy for every other party to the proceedings.

4. Before you answer Yes to Question 5 you should understand that:-

    (a) If the petitioner satisfies the court that the petitioner and you have been living apart for two years immediately before the presentation of the petition and that you consent to a decree, the Court will grant one unless it considers that the marriage has not broken down irretrievably.

    (b) A decree absolute of divorce will end your marriage so that:-

        (i) any right you may have to a pension which depends on the marriage continuing will be affected;

        (ii) you will not be able to claim a State Widow's pension when the petitioner dies;

        (iii) any rights of occupation you may have in the matrimonial home under the Matrimonial Homes Act 1983 will cease unless the Court has ordered otherwise before the decree is granted;

    (c) Once the Court grants a decree absolute or decree of judicial separation, you will lose your right to inherit from the petitioner if he or she dies without having made a will, and if the petitioner has made a will a decree absolute of divorce will deprive you of any right which you may have under that will to act as executor or to take any gift under the will, unless a contrary intention appears in the will.

    (d) A decree may have other consequences in your case depending on your particular circumstances and if you are in any doubt about these you would be well advised to consult a solicitor.

5. If after consenting you wish to withdraw your consent you must immediately inform the Court and give notice to the solicitor.

6. If you answer Yes to Question 6 you must before the decree is made absolute, make application to the Court by filing and serving on the petitioner a notice in form **D64** which may be obtained from the Court.

7. (a) If you do not wish to defend the case but object to the claim for costs, you should answer Yes to Question 7 in the acknowledgement. You must state the grounds on which you object. An objection cannot be entertained unless the grounds are given which, if established, would form a valid reason for not paying the costs. If such grounds are given, you will be notified of a date on which you must attend before the Judge if you wish to pursue the objection.

   (b) If you do not object to the claim for costs but simply wish to be heard on the amount to be allowed, you should answer No to Question 7.

   (c) If you are ordered to pay costs, the amount will be assessed by the Court unless it is agreed between the petitioner and yourself or fixed at a prescribed sum. If costs are to be assessed, you will be sent a copy of the petitioner's bill of costs and will have the right to be heard about the amount before it is finally settled.

8. (a) Please answer Question 8.
   If your answer to Question 8(c) is Yes please make sure that you sign the form at 10(a)

9. If you wish to contest the petitioner's financial or property claim, you will have an opportunity of doing so when you receive a notice stating that the petitioner intends to proceed with the claim. You will then be required to file an affidavit giving particulars of your property and income and be notified of the date when the claim is to be heard.

10. If you wish to make some financial or property claim on your own account, you will have to make a separate application. If you are in doubt as to the consequences of divorce on your financial position, you should obtain legal advice from a solicitor.

11. If you wish to make an order for:-

   * a Residence Order
   * a Contact Order
   * a Specific Issue Order
   * a Prohibited Steps Order

   in respect of a child, you will have to make a separate application on form CHA 10(D). You can get this form from the Court Office. Before you apply for any of these orders or for any other orders which may be available to you under Part I or II of the Children Act ·you are advised to see a solicitor.

Dated 14 February 1994

Address all communications for the court to the Principal Registry of the Family Division, Family Proceedings Department, Somerset House, Strand, London WC2R 1LP AND QUOTE THE ABOVE CASE NUMBER. The Court Office at the Principal Registry is open from 10am till 4.30pm, on Mondays to Fridays.

Notice of Proceedings – Respondent Spouse
MCA 1973 – Section 1(2) (A)(b)(c)
F.P. Rule 2.6 (6)

In the PRINCIPAL REGISTRY

No. of Matter 3554

Between   Alice Jane Roberts   Petitioner

and Ronald James Roberts   Respondent

and   Co-Respondent

- If you intend to instruct a solicitor to act for you, give him this form immediately
- Read carefully the Notice of Proceedings before answering the following questions
- Please complete using black ink

1. Have you received the petition for divorce delivered with this form?	Yes
2. On which date and at what address did you receive it?	On the 20th day of February 1994 at Flat 9 Cherrytree Gardens Meadstown
3. Are you the person named as the Respondent in the petition?	Yes
4. Do you intend to defend the case?	No
5. Do you consent to a decree being granted?	Yes
6. In the event of a decree nisi being granted on the basis of two years' separation coupled with the respondent's consent, do you intend to apply to the Court for it to consider your financial position as it will be after the divorce?	Yes
7. Even if you do not intend to defend the case do you object to paying the costs of the proceedings? If so, on what grounds?	No
8. (a) Have you received a copy of the Statement of Arrangements for the child(ren)?	(a) Yes
(b) What was the date of the Statement of Arrangements? (the date beside the Petitioner's signature at Part 3)	(b) 15 February
(c) Do you agree with the proposals in that Statement of Arrangements? Notes If NO you may file a written Statement of your views on the present and the proposed arrangements for the children. It would help if you sent that Statement to the court office with this form. You can get a form from the court office	(c) Yes
9. *(In the case of proceedings relating to a polygamous marriage)* If you have any wife/husband in addition to the petitioner who is not mentioned in the petition, what is the name and address of each such wife/husband and the date and place of your marriage to her/him?	N/A

10(a). You must complete this part if

    * you answered Yes to Question 5

    or

    * you answered Yes to Question 8(c)

    or

    * you do not have a solicitor acting for you

    Signed: R J Roberts   Date: 25 March 1994

    Address for service: as above

    *Note: If you are acting on your own you should also put your place of residence, or if you do not reside in England or Wales the address of a place in England or Wales to which documents may be sent to you. If you subsequently wish to change your address for service, you must notify the court.

10(b) I am/We are acting for the Respondent in this matter.

    Signed: Clements & Co   Solicitor(s) for the Respondent

    Date: 1st April 1994

    Address for service:

        75 High Street Meadstown

    Note: If your client answered **Yes** to Question 5 or Question 8(c) **your client must sign and date at 10(a)**

Address all communications for the Court to the Chief Clerk **and quote the above case number** The Court Office at

        The Principal Registry
        of the Family Division
        Somerset House, Strand
        WC2R 1LP

        is open from 10am to 4.30pm on Monday to Fridays only

Acknowledgement of Service – Respondent spouse

F.P. Rule 2.9(5) (Form M6)

Form M7(d) in Appendix 1 to the Family
Proceedings Rules 1991

SPECIMEN

Affidavit by petitioner in support of petition under
section 1(2)(d) of Matrimonial Causes Act 1973

2 YEARS SEPARATION AND CONSENT

IN THE   **COUNTY COURT***

No. of matter 3554 of 94

Between   Alice Jane Roberts   Petitioner

and
          Ronald James Roberts   Respondent

QUESTION	ANSWER
About the Divorce Petition 1 Have you read the petition filed in this case?	Yes
2 Do you wish to alter or add to any statement in the petition? If so, state the alterations or additions	No
3 Subject to these alterations and additions (if any), is everything stated in your petition true? If any statement is not within your own knowledge, indicate this and say whether it is true to the best of your information and belief.	Yes
4 State the date on which you and the respondent separated.	31st January 1992
5 State briefly the reason or main reason for the separation.	We were unable to resolve our differences
6 State the date when and the circumstances in which you came to the conclusion that marriage was in fact at an end.	15th January 1992 after a long discussion with the Respondent

7 State as far as you know the various addresses at which you and the respondent have respectively lived since the date given in the answer to Question 4, and the periods of residence at each

Petitioner's Address   Respondent's Address

From   From
31.1.93 5 Woodside Meadstown   31.1.93   Flat 9 Cherrytree
to the present   to the present Gardens Meadstown

8 Since the date given in the answer to Question 4, have you ever lived with the respondent in the same household? If so, state the address and the period or periods, giving dates.	No

About the children of the family

9 Have you read the Statement of Arrangements filed in this case?	Yes
10 Do you wish to alter anything in the Statement of Arrangements or add to it? If so, state the alterations or additions.	No
11 Subject to these alterations and addition(s) (if any) is everything stated in your petition [and Statement of Arrangements for the child(ren)] true and correct to the best of your knowledge and belief?	Yes

I, Alice Jane Roberts   (full name)

of 5 Woodside Meadstown Beamshire   (full residential address)

School teacher   (occupation)

make oath and say as follows:

1   I am the petitioner in this cause.

2   **The answers to Questions 1 to 11 above are true.**

(1) Insert name of the respondent exactly as it appears in the acknowledgement of service signed by him/her.

3(1) I identify the signature ...... R. J. Roberts .... (1) appearing on the copy acknowledgment of service now produced to me and marked 'A' as the signature of my husband/wife, the respondent in this cause.

4   I identify the signature .... (1) appearing at Part IV of the Statement of Arrangements dated .... now produced and shown to me and marked 'B' as the signature of the respondent.

(2)Exhibit any other document on which the petitioner wishes to reply.

5(2)

(3)If the petitioner seeks a judicial separation amend accordingly.

6   I ask the court to grant a decree dissolving my marriage with the respondent(3) on the grounds stated in my petition [and to order the respondent to pay the costs of this suit](4)

(4)Delete if costs are not sought.

Sworn at 7 Laurel Avenue   )
Meadstown   )   A.J. Roberts
in the County of Beamshire)........................

this 6th day of May 1994)
Before me ...... A. Turney ....
A Commissioner for Oaths.
Officer of the court appointed
(5)Delete as the case may be.
by the Judge to take affidavits(5)

IN THE PRINCIPAL REGISTRY

No. 3554 of 1994

Between
    Alice Jane Roberts
                Petitioner

and
    Ronald James Roberts
                Respondent

Affidavit by petitioner
in support of petition
under section 1(2)(d)
of the Matrimonial
Causes Act 1973

Grossfees & Co
75 High Street
Meadstown
Beamshire

Solicitors for the Petitioner

Application for Directions for Trial (Special Procedure)

| SPECIMEN |

FAMILY PROCEEDINGS   No.   **3554 of 1994**
RULES (Rule 2.24)   **IN THE PRINCIPAL REGISTRY**

Between   Alice Jane Roberts   Petitioner

and   Ronald James Roberts   Respondent

Application for Directions for Trial (Special Procedure)

The Petitioner   Alice Jane Roberts

applies to the District Judge for directions for the trial of this undefended
cause by entering it in the Special Procedure List.

The Petitioner's affidavit of evidence is lodged with this application.

Signed   Grossfees & Co   [Solicitors for] the Petitioner

Dated   10th May 1994

If you write to the Court please address your letters to 'The Chief Clerk'

and quote the **No. of Matter** at the top of this form.

The Principal Registry is at Somerset House, Strand, London WC2R 1LP

and is open from 10 am to 4.30 pm on Monday to Friday.

Divorce 51B

```
┌─────────────┐
│ SPECIMEN    │    Special Procedure: Directions for Trial
└─────────────┘
```

No. 3554 of 1994

PRINCIPAL REGISTRY OF THE FAMILY DIVISION

Between	Roberts, Alice Jane	Petitioner
and	Roberts, Ronald James	Respondent
and		

DIRECTIONS FOR TRIAL

I am satisfied that the requirements of Rules 2.24(1) and 2.24(3) have been complied with, and I direct that this cause be entered in the County/High Court Special Procedure List.

(a) the Respondent's   adultery [with
(b) the Respondent's   unreasonable behaviour]
(c) the Respondent's   2 years' desertion
(d) 2 years' separation and consent
(e) 5 years' separation

---

*   and to an order that the
    do pay
    the costs of the Petitioner

---

*   and to an order for ancillary relief as agreed between the Petitioner
    and Respondent.

---

*   and I further certify that I am satisfied that there are no children
    to whom section 41 of the Matrimonial Causes Act 1973 applies

---

*   Delete the boxes which do not apply

Date: 18th July 1994   District Judge A. A. Gabriel

TAKE NOTICE that the Court has fixed
the 8th day of August 1994 at 10.30am
[for the pronouncement of a decree] [and the making of the orders
included in the District Judge's Certificate] by a

[District Judge sitting at the Principal Registry of the Family
Division, Somerset House, Strand, London WC2R 1LP]

[Judge sitting at the Royal Courts of Justice, Strand, London, WC2A 2LL]

*Note: unless the decree or any of the orders is opposed, it is
unnecessary for any party to appear at Court for the pronouncement.*

IMPORTANT: If there are children of the family please see overleaf
for further details

This section to be completed only if Directions for Trial have been given and where the application is pending under Parts I or II of the Children Act 1989 in relation to the child(ren) of the family

2. CHILDREN DIRECTION

I certify that I am satisfied that there [is a] [are] child(ren) of the family to whom section 41 of the Matrimonial Causes Act 1973 applies

> * [but the court does not need to exercise its powers under the Children Act 1989 with respect to [any of them] [that child]]
> [nor give any direction under section 41(2) of the Matrimonial Causes Act 1973]

I am not satisfied because

and I direct that

> * (a) for the following child(ren):
>
> the [Petitioner][Respondent] [the following person(s)]
>
> shall attend before District Judge
>
> in Room , Principal Registry of the Family Division, Somerset House, Strand, London WC2R 1LP,
>
> on day, the day of 19
>
> at am/pm
> [for a conciliation appointment]
> [when the Court will consider the arrangements for the child(ren)]

> * (b) for the following child(ren):
>
> a welfare report shall be prepared by

> * (c) for the following child(ren)
>
> the [Petitioner] [Respondent] [the following person(s)]
>
> shall file further evidence [specifically on]

> * (d) for the following children

> * (e) the decree shall not be made absolute until the Court orders otherwise [because]

* Delete the boxes which do not apply
Date: 18th July 1994   A. A. Gabriel   District Judge

Address all communications for the Court to the Principal Registry of the Family Division, Family Proceedings Department, Somerset House, Strand, London WC2R 1LP, quoting the number in the top right hand corner of this form. The court office is open from 10.00 am until 4.30 pm on Mondays to Fridays.

Notice of making Decree Nisi

No 3554 of 1994

List No.

IN THE HIGH COURT OF JUSTICE
PRINCIPAL REGISTRY OF THE FAMILY DIVISION

Matrimonial cause proceeding in the Principal Registry by virtue of section 42 of the Matrimonial and Family Proceedings Act 1984 as pending in a divorce county court

(Before His Honour Judge
sitting at the Royal Courts of Justice, Strand, London)

(Before Mr   District Judge A.A. Gabriel
sitting at the Principal Registry of the Family Division, Somerset House, Strand, London)

Between	Alice Jane Roberts	Petitioner
and	Ronald James Roberts	Respondent
and		Co-Respondent

On the 8th day of August 1994

the (District) Judge held

that the marriage solemnised

on the 15th day of March 1972

at The Register Office Crowbury Dorset

between	Alice Jane Roberts	Petitioner
and	Ronald James Roberts	Respondent

has broken down irretrievably and decreed that the said marriage be dissolved unless sufficient cause be shown to the court within six weeks from the making of this decree why such decree should not be made absolute.

THIS IS NOT THE FINAL DECREE
Application for this decree to be made absolute must be made not earlier than six weeks from the above date.

Address all communications for the Court to the Principal Registry of the Family Division, Family Proceedings Department, Somerset House, Strand, London WC2R 1LP quoting the number in the top right hand corner of this form. The Court Office at the Principal Registry is open from 10.00am until 4.30pm on Mondays to Fridays.

Orders on making Decree Nisi

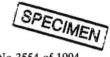

No 3554 of 1994
List No.

IN THE HIGH COURT OF JUSTICE

PRINCIPAL REGISTRY OF THE FAMILY DIVISION

Matrimonial cause proceeding in the Principal Registry by virtue of section 42 of the Matrimonial and Family Proceedings Act 1984 as pending in a divorce county court

[Before   His Honour Judge
sitting at the Royal Courts of Justice, Strand, London]

[Before   Mr District Judge Gabriel
sitting at the Principal Registry of the Family Division, Strand, London]

Between   ALICE JANE ROBERTS
Petitioner

and   RONALD JAMES ROBERTS
Respondent

and
Co-Respondent

On the 8th day of August 1994

upon the making of the Decree Nisi herein it is ordered that the

respondent

do pay the costs incurred and to be incurred on behalf of the Petitioner in this cause.

[And it is declared that the Court is satisfied that, for the purposes of section 41 of the Matrimonial Causes Act 1973, there are no children of the family to whom the said section applies.]

Address all communications for the Court to the Principal Registry of the Family Division, Family Proceedings Department, Somerset House, Strand, London WC2R 1LP quoting the number in the top right hand corner of this form. The Principal Registry is open from 10.00am until 4.30pm on Mondays to Fridays.

Notice of making Decree Nisi Absolute (Divorce) ⌈SPECIMEN⌉

No. 3554 of 1994

IN THE COURT OF JUSTICE
PRINCIPAL REGISTRY OF THE FAMILY DIVISION
Matrimonial cause proceedings in Principal Registry treated by
virtue of section 42 of the Matrimonial and Family Proceedings
Act 1984 as pending in a divorce county court

Between	ALICE JANE ROBERTS	Petitioner
and	RONALD JAMES ROBERTS	Respondent
and		Co-Respondent

Referring to the decree made in this cause

on the   8th   day of August   1994

whereby it was decreed that the marriage solemnised

on the   15th   day of March   1972

at The Register Office Crowbury Dorset

between the petitioner and the respondent be dissolved unless sufficient
case be shown to the court within
six weeks from the making thereof why the said decree should not be
made absolute, and no cause having been shown, it is hereby certified that
the said decree was

on the   30th   day of March   1995

made final and absolute and that the said marriage was thereby dissolved.

Dated this   30th   day of March   1995

Note Divorce affects inheritance under a will.

Where a will has already been made by either party to the marriage
then, by virtue of section 18A of the Wills Act 1837, from the above date
on which the decree was made absolute:-

(a) any appointment of the former spouse as an executor or

trustee is treated as if omitted;

and

(b) any gift in the will to the former spouse lapses;

unless a contrary intention appears in the will.

**Address all communications to the Principal Registry of the Family
Division, Family Proceedings Department, Somerset House, Strand,
London WC2R 1LP quoting the number in the top right hand corner of
this form. The Principal Registry is open from 10.00am until 4.30pm
Mondays to Fridays.**

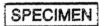

Notice of Application for Ancillary Relief (Agreed terms)
(Form M11, Appendix 1, F.P.R. 1991)

FAMILY PROCEEDINGS RULES
Rule 2.53(2) and (3)
*Compete and/or delete as appropriate. If proceeding in a District Registry, delete both headings and insert 'In the High Court of Justice, Family Division, District Registry'.

(1) Petitioner or Respondent.
(2) Here set out the ancillary relief claimed, stating the terms of any agreement as to the order which the court is to be asked to make, and in the case of an application for a property adjustment order or an avoidance of disposition order, stating briefly the nature of the adjustment proposed or the disposition to be set aside. If the application is to **vary** periodical payments of secured periodical payments for **children**, state here whether there are or have been any proceedings in the Child Support Agency relating to their maintenance.

(3) Delete whichever is not applicable.

(4) Delete this line and insert the appropriate address in the line above if this application is not proceeding in the Principal Registry.

(5)Unless the parties are agreed upon the terms of the proposed order, or the application is for a variation order, add:

IN THE _____ **COUNTY COURT***
PRINCIPAL REGISTRY*
No. of Matter

Between .... A.J. Roberts .... .Petitioner
and .... R.J. Roberts .... .Respondent
[and ....Co-respondent]
Take Notice that the Petitioner   intends to apply to the Court for(^{2})

If you are applying for any periodical payments or secured periodical payments for **children**, please say here whether you are applying for payment ☐ for a stepchild or step children ☐ in addition to child support maintenance already paid under a Child Support Agency assessment ☐ to meet expenses arising from a child's disability ☐ to meet expenses incurred by a child in being educated or training for work ☐ when either the child **OR** the person with care of the child, **OR** the absent parent of the child is not habitually resident in the United Kingdom ☐ other (please specify).

(^{3})Notice will be given to you of the place and time fixed for the hearing of the application
OR
(^{3})The application will be heard by the District Judge in chambers at
on   day, the   day of   , 19   , at   o'clock.
OR
(^{4}) at Room   , the Principal Registry, Somerset House, Strand, London WC2R 1LP,
on   day, the   day of   , 19   , at   o'clock.
The probable length of the hearing of this application is

(^{5}) **Take Notice also that** you must send to the district judge, so as to reach him/her within 28 days after you receive a copy of the affidavit of the Petitioner [or Respondent], an affidavit giving full particulars of your property and income. You must at the same time sent a copy of your affidavit to [the solicitor for] the applicant.
A standard form of affidavit may be obtained from the Court Office.
If you wish to allege that the(^{1})
has property or income, you should say so in your affidavit.
Dated this   day of   19

(*Signed*) .Grossfees.&.Co .... Solicitors for the(^{1}).Petitioner
of......................
....
Address all communications for the Court to: The Chief Clerk, County Court* ....
....

(or to the Principal Registry, Somerset House, Strand, London WC2R 1LP) quoting the number in the top right-hand corner of this form.
This Court Office is open from 10 a.m. till 4 p.m. (4.30 p.m. at the Principal Registry) on Mondays to Fridays only.

Affidavit sworn 15 March 1995
exhibits

IN THE PRINCIPAL REGISTRY   **No. 3554 of 1994**

BETWEEN

ALICE JANE ROBERTS

Petitioner

and

RONALD JAMES ROBERTS

Respondent

**AFFIDAVIT OF MEANS OF THE PETITIONER
IN SUPPORT OF HER APPLICATION FOR
ANCILLARY RELIEF**

I Alice Jane Roberts of 5 Woodside, Meadstown, Beamshire the
Petitioner herein MAKE OATH and say as follows:-

1. I am 39 years of age and was married to the Respondent who is
now 44 on the 15 March 1972. There are two sons of our marriage,
David now aged 16 and John who is 13. The decree nisi was
pronounced on the 8 August 1994.

2. I met the Respondent in London when I was teaching immediately after leaving university. He taught evening classes in wood-
work which I attended because of my interest in carpentry. The
Respondent was also interested in painting and enjoyed going to
galleries. As a student of French I had taken a particular interest in
the history of French painting. We married within six months.

3. We lived initially in a rented flat but both of us were keen to
acquire a home of our own and have children so that when less
than two years later an appropriate job became available in a large
comprehensive school in Meadstown we decided that the
Respondent should apply for it. He was successful, I gave up my
job and we moved to our previous matrimonial home 31 Lukes

Terrace three months before David's birth. The house cost £25,000, Respondent had savings of £1,500 and I had £500. My parents loaned us £1,000 and we obtained a mortgage for £24,000. It was supported by a with profits endowment policy in our joint names with Lifelong Insurance Company.

4. We sold 31 Lukes Terrace for £40,000 nine years ago after making considerable improvements to it. The Respondent had built a conservatory largely through his own efforts and with the help of a friend and the cost of the materials and some payment to the friend was met by a bank loan which was repaid. The present house 5 Woodside was bought for £130,000. The net proceeds of sale of the first house were £12,000. The Respondent had inherited money when his parents had died and that amounted to approximately £75,000 of which £60,000 was put into the house. I do not know what happened to the balance. We again obtained a mortgage this time of £60,000 collaterally secured with the former endowment policy and a further endowment policy with the same company for £36,000 on our joint lives. The property was bought in our joint names on a joint tenancy basis. I have served notice of severance to create a tenancy in common because I am not satisfied that if I died first and the Respondent inherited it he would provide by will for our sons.

5. Considerable work has been done to the property both structural and decorative. A new central heating system was installed and the decorating was done to a high standard. When the recession began to affect the Respondent's business four years ago he obtained a floating charge for his company from the bank. I was advised that I should seek independent advice before signing the charge. Regrettably, I did not do so. I believed and still believe in the Respondent's ability to repay it or alternatively to secure it on the freehold factory building which I believe is not now currently fully charged. In any event, I do not accept that it should be taken account of in deciding the extent of the equity of the house. I put the Respondent to full proof of the current extent of the charge.

6. Six years ago we bought for £25,000 a cottage in the Western Highlands of Scotland. It was funded entirely by the Respondent who had a large income that year. The property was bought in our joint names. It was a solid building but had and has no central heating. The Respondent has made improvements to it and we have

used it for holidays at Easter and in the summer and occasionally for weekends but given the expense of air fares this has not been possible since the separation. The property is probably worth about £30,000.

7. 5 Woodside has four good sized bedrooms, two bathrooms and a large garden. It is a suitable home for me and our sons and I would not want to be forced to sell it. Our sons have already had a sufficiently disturbing time during the last two years and I am anxious to provide some stability for them at least during their remaining years at school.

8. I earn £25,000 as Head of the French Department at Gregsons School, the same school at which the Respondent obtained his first job here. My net salary is £1548.73 per month. I put £1,000 into our joint account each month with Gribbins Bank. The Respondent while he was at home used to put £2,000 per month into it but this has now been reduced to £1,200. The balance of my salary goes into my sole account with the same bank. I use my account for the purchase of personal items for myself including my clothes, clothes for the boys and household items such as soft furnishings. I have over the years made a lot of the curtains and soft furnishings in the house as well as undertaking occasional decorating and this has saved us a good deal of money which was of particular importance when the business was being established.

9. A year before we bought our present house the Respondent and his brother began a light engineering firm producing spare parts for the motor industry. Initially I was company secretary and for some three years received a salary. That then ceased. My brother-in-law contributed some capital to the company. My husband bought a freehold factory on the outskirts of the town. The business expanded and became very successful partly because it was economically run with the most modern machinery. The Respondent's earnings gave us a very comfortable standard of living. I appreciate that the scale of the business has now reduced and with some staff cuts has resulted in lower production but I believe that it will recover and that the present debt level will not remain.

10. Our marriage began to deteriorate about four years ago after my husband had formed an increasingly close friendship with

Arthur Walker a successful artist now aged 55. He spent a good deal of time going to exhibitions in London with Arthur but it was some time before I realised the true nature of their relationship. It was not something to which I wished to refer in my Petition but its relevance to our financial futures is clear. The children were initially very disturbed by the situation and I cannot judge what its long-term effects on them may be. The Respondent moved out two years ago and has since shared Arthur Walker's flat. Contact with the children has been regular subject to their weekend activities and they go away for holidays with the Respondent in the summer and at Christmas.

11. My financial future is far from secure. Thankfully as Head of a department I am unlikely to be sacked in the staff cuts now being imposed but future pay increases are unlikely to be dramatic and I may have to take early retirement. I will have a modest pension on retirement. If the marriage had continued I would have expected provision from my husband's self-administered pension scheme; although I am not a member of it I would have shared the benefits of his pension income. The pension fund has a current value of £250,000 I believe. While I do not seek maintenance for myself I ask that my maintenance rights are not dismissed. I seek a lump sum based on the equity in the house disregarding the charge for the benefit of the company together with the other available assets. If as I understand it I am not entitled to any share in the company's assets I think it is wrong that I should be expected to share in responsibility for its debts. But I do maintain that I should not live in the future in circumstances reduced by the fact of a divorce which I did not want. If my needs warrant it I think that later on I should be able to claim maintenance. I therefore ask for nominal maintenance. I shall have no private health insurance which I have had in the past and I shall have needs from time to time such as a replacement car. The present one a Vauxhall saloon belongs to the company and is worth about £6,000. I have no plans to remarry. The Respondent has made much of a relationship I have had with David Mitchem a divorced colleague of 35 with two young children. I do not intend to live with him nor to marry him.

12. On the question of maintenance for the children we are agreed that the Respondent will pay £7,000 per annum in respect

of David and John. Additionally, he will pay the school fees of David who will attend a fee-paying school for his sixth form years. This decision was agreed by us in view of the fact that my own school which he currently attends with the forthcoming reduction in staff cannot offer the same opportunities for advanced levels as a local fee-paying school, Haydens. We have not agreed what would be appropriate for John because it is premature to make such a decision while he is only 13.

13. My current monthly outgoings are as follows:

Household expenses

Food including entertaining at home, occasional restaurant	£600.00
Gas	50.00
Electricity	65.00
Telephone	60.00
Chemist, cosmetics, dental, optical charges	50.00
Maintenance, repairs and replacement of household items	50.00
TV licence and rental	75.00

Travel

Fares (boys £10.00 per week)	44.00
Train costs	165.00
Holidays	200.00

Motoring expenses

Road tax	10.83
Insurance	40.00
Petrol	120.00

Insurances

Structural insurance and contents insurance premiums	85.00
Mortgage	350.00

Personal expenses

Clothes – mine	125.00
Clothes – children's	100.00
Books, magazines, subscriptions	45.00
Birthday and Christmas presents	125.00
	£2,359.83

14. My assets apart from my share in the matrimonial home and Hillside the Scottish property consist of a Tessa account with Beamshire Building Society with £5,800 and jewellery worth £5,000 which is not insured. I put the Respondent to full proof of his assets. I believe that apart from the company in which he has a 95% share whose value I am advised by my accountant and believe from his study of the 1994 accounts to be worth about £300,000 including the real value of the freehold land. I am confident in his ability to develop the business in better circumstances. I do not seek to make his borrowing position more difficult but ask the court to accept that the charge on the house should not be debited against the family capital. I believe that the Respondent has some investments but I do not know of what they consist. I ask the court to award me such maintenance and capital as may be just.

SWORN by the said ALICE JANE ROBERTS)
this   15th   day of   March 1995   )
at   )

Before me,

A Solicitor

Affidavit
sworn February 1995
exhibits

IN THE PRINCIPAL REGISTRY
No. 3554 of 1994

BETWEEN

ALICE JANE ROBERTS
Petitioner
and

RONALD JAMES ROBERTS
Respondent

**AFFIDAVIT OF MEANS OF THE
PETITIONER IN SUPPORT OF HER
APPLICATION FOR ANCILLARY
RELIEF**

1st Affidavit of Respondent
sworn   1995
exhibits

IN THE PRINCIPAL REGISTRY   **No. 3554 of 1994**

BETWEEN

ALICE JANE ROBERTS

                                                 Petitioner

and

RONALD JAMES ROBERTS

                                                 Respondent

AFFIDAVIT OF MEANS OF THE RESPONDENT

I RONALD JAMES ROBERTS of Flat 9 Cherrytree Gardens, Meadstown, Beamshire the Respondent herein **MAKE OATH** and say as follows:-

1. I have read a copy of the Affidavit sworn by the Petitioner on the 15 March 1995 and make this my Affidavit in Reply. I begin by placing on record the fact that I greatly regret the pain I have caused the Petitioner and the confusion to my children by my new relationship and I acknowledge that the Petitioner has enabled me to maintain my relationship with our sons in very difficult circumstances. The numbers of the paragraphs which follow bear the same number of those in the Petitioner's affidavit to which I am responding.

(3) The Petitioner omits to mention that when I began my business a year before we sold our first house I had obtained a charge secured on that house for a loan of £15,000 to the bank. The reason for this was that I was re-equipping the factory I had bought and its freehold value was inadequate security for all my borrowings.

(4) and (7) After my parents' death I used £15,000 to repay the

charge. The implication of what the Petitioner says is that I used the balance of my inheritance for other purposes. The other figures are correctly stated. The two endowment policies now have a surrender value worth £30,000 with 16 years for the one to run and 10 years for the other. I was sorry that the Petitioner severed the joint tenancy of our former home. I would wish her to have the house if I died and since she has severed the tenancy I have made a new will leaving her my share or if she does not survive me, our sons. The charge to Gribbins Bank which is secured on the house is about £50,000. I was not aware that the Petitioner had failed to take independent advice as recommended by the bank before she signed the charge. She has been happy to share the benefits of my work in better times but is reluctant to accept that the present reality is that the equity in the house is diminished by the charge and that a sale is the only way at present of repaying it. The house is worth probably £250,000 and the building society mortgage which is not a repayment mortgage is £60,000. I have no wish to disturb my sons' occupation of it but I believe it will be possible to buy an acceptable replacement home for £135,000 and the net equity would provide sufficient for them to do this and pay the associated removal costs.

(6) Our cottage in Scotland should probably be sold to provide much-needed cash. There is unlikely to be any capital gains tax involved.

(8) It is true that I have reduced my contribution to the account but the Petitioner overlooks the fact that I put £100 per month into savings accounts for David and John and that my absence from the house means that her overall expenditure does not have to provide for me. I also have outgoings as a result of my move. I pay Arthur Walker £250 per month towards my keep and overheads. I have bought items such as folding beds for the boys at the flat I share with Arthur Walker and I have bought items for the boys such as sports equipment from time to time. There is no need for me to pay £2,000 per month into the account. It is currently in credit. At the agreed level of maintenance to the boys I will be paying £583 per month for them. Even if the family stayed in the former matrimonial home it will be a long time before any significant repairs or maintenance were needed but as I have said it should be sold and should certainly attract a price of about £250,000.

(9) My brother who has a very successful retail business gave me a substantial loan to start the business. I was helped by a bank mortgage on the factory premises. During the 1980s the business grew until I had 100 staff. As demand shrank I could not afford to maintain the former scale of production and reduced my staff to 75. The Petitioner was fully aware how the business ran because as she herself points out she was a secretary in the early days. She was also a shareholder with 1% but I bought this share for £5,000 which enabled her to put it into the building society.

(10) My present accommodation is in Arthur Walker's studio flat which is worth no more than £45,000. It is too cramped for our occupation. I need a house with two or three bedrooms in which the boys can stay. So far as my future plans are concerned I intend to continue living with Arthur Walker. His financial future is far from secure. I mention this fact because although I do not support him I am conscious that he suffers from arthritis which already impairs his ability to paint. He has some small income from inherited capital.

(11) I am hopeful that my business will recover but do not think it will reach its former levels. The Petitioner has already seen the 1994 accounts and I am happy to give her full discovery. The company is now worth £200,000 including the value of the factory freehold. I have a self-administered pension fund worth £250,000. It is true that if the marriage continued the Petitioner would share in the income it will generate for my retirement. The only way in which I could enable her to benefit from it would be by having a defined share of the lump sum element which would be payable to me on my retirement. Of course this amount is not ascertainable at present. I am advised that the court cannot order me to make provision from my pension fund for the Petitioner although it can order me to pay a particular lump sum at a particular time but I am happy that depending upon the other awards made to her and on the basis that there is a clean break in relation to maintenance that she should have one quarter of the sum which I receive by way of lump sum or £25,000 whichever may be the larger. Expressed in this way it means that I would have some freedom to choose between a larger and a smaller lump sum because that would affect the amount of pension I would thereafter receive and I would not want to have a diminished pension because of an obligation to pay an unrealistically high amount of lump sum to the Petitioner. I

would however, not be happy for such a lump sum to be paid to the Petitioner if she had at that stage remarried. I am also happy to provide on the same basis that she should be the beneficiary from my death in service provision which would ensure that she would have money for herself and more important the children should I die before the age of 60. She is in any event the beneficiary of my life policy. I have noted what the Petitioner says of her intentions in relation to David Mitchem but do not necessarily expect that her views will remain unchanged. The overall assets position at present is as follows:

5 Woodside		£250,000.00	
Less mortgage	60,000.00		
Bank charge	50,000.00	110,000.00	£140,000.00

Surrender values of policies with Lifelong	
Insurance Co.	30,000.00
Scottish property	30,000.00
My personal equity plans	20,000.00
Petitioner's Tessa	5,800.00
Petitioner's jewellery	5,000.00
Surrender value of life policy	35,000.00
	£265,800.00

Note

I have not included in the above figures the transfer value of my pension fund which is as already set out £250,000 nor the value of the company which is worth approximately £200,000. I am happy that the Petitioner should have on a clean-break basis the net equity of the two properties and to have the endowment policies transferred into her sole name. That would give her with her personal assets all the available assets save for my PEPS worth £20,000. Additionally, she would benefit from my life policy if she survived me and if she had not remarried would have the protection of my death in service provision if I were to die in service otherwise on my retirement she would receive a lump sum of £25,000.

(12) I confirm my agreement. I am hopeful that we shall also be able to agree on John's future education.

(13) I believe that in the smaller but still suitable house the maintenance and fuel costs would be considerably reduced. If the Petitioner has the Scottish property she can sell it or pending sale derive income from it; she should be able to receive some rent after tax is paid.

SWORN by the said **RONALD JAMES ROBERTS**)
this 5th day of May 1995   )
at 75 High Street, Meadstown   )

Before me,

A Solicitor

Affidavit sworn
February 1995
exhibits

IN THE PRINCIPAL REGISTRY
No. 3554 of 1994

BETWEEN

ALICE JANE ROBERTS
                    Petitioner
and

RONALD JAMES ROBERTS

                    Respondent

AFFIDAVIT OF MEANS OF THE RESPONDENT

IN THE PRINCIPAL REGISTRY   No. 3554 of 1994

BETWEEN

ALICE JANE ROBERTS

Petitioner

and

RONALD JAMES ROBERTS

Respondent

REPLIES TO QUESTIONNAIRE OF THE PETITIONER
SERVED ON 15 APRIL 1995 DATED 6 JUNE 1995

Question

Bank and Building Society accounts

1. A schedule of all (current, deposit, loan or other) bank accounts which the Respondent has held in his sole name, jointly with any other person(s) or by his nominee(s), or in which he has had any beneficial interest, whether in the United Kingdom or anywhere else in the world, during the last three years.

Reply

The Respondent has three accounts at Gribbins Bank:

(I) Sole account number 0257934

(ii) Joint account with brother number 0426735

(iii) Company account Roberts Engineering Limited number 09146297

Question

2. A schedule of all building society or other savings or deposit accounts (not covered by Paragraph 1 above) which the Respondent has held in his sole name, jointly with any other person(s) or by his nominee(s), or in which he has had any beneficial interest, whether in the United Kingdom or anywhere else in the world, during the last three years.

Reply

The Respondent has none.

Question

3. Copy statements/pass sheets relating to all accounts referred to in Paragraphs 1 and 2 above in respect of the period from December 1994 to the date of answering this Questionnaire, and continuing thereafter to the date of trial unless the Petitioner's Solicitors give notice to the contrary.

Reply

Attached herewith in relation to three above accounts.

Question

4. Identification of all credit entries appearing in the said statements/pass sheets in excess of £500 and all debit entries in excess of £500.

Reply

This is oppressive particularly with respect to the company account.

Correspondence with Bankers

Question

5. Copies of all correspondence passing between the Respondent or his Accountants on the one hand and his Bankers (or any of them) on the other hand during the last three years with regard to the bank charge on the former matrimonial home.

Reply

Herewith letter from Bank dated 3 June 1991 and copy letter enclosed with it to the Petitioner advising her to obtain independent advice.

Question

Cohabitee: dispositions to

6. Has the Respondent made any financial dispositions, in cash or in kind, to Arthur Walker? If so, please give full particulars, disclosing any documents relating thereto in the custody, possession or power of the Respondent and identifying any relevant entry in the Respondent's bank or building society statements/pass sheets.

Reply

No, save as disclosed monthly payments of £250 by way of rent.

Question

Cohabitee: means of

7. To the best of the knowledge, information and belief of the Respondent, what are the means and other relevant circumstances of Arthur Walker?

Reply

They are as disclosed. I belive his capital to be in the region of £75,000 and income derived from investments about £3,000.

Question

Company (private): accounts and other information

8. As to the company Roberts Engineering Limited ('the Company'):
   (a) Copies of the Accounts of the Company (if necessary in draft) for the year ended 31.3.95
   (b) If the Accounts of the Company for the year ended 31.3.95 are not yet available, even in draft, when is it expected that their preparation will be completed? A letter from the Company's Accountants explaining the position is requested.
   (c) Copies of any existing Management Accounts in respect of the period from the date of the last accounts provided in answer to (a) above to the date of answering this Questionnaire.
   (d) As to the Accounts of the Company for the year ended 31.3.94 already disclosed by the Respondent
      (i) Have there been any and if so what professional valuations of the land and factory buildings in question during the last three years? If so, please produce copies of the same and in any event what is the Respondent's estimate of the open market value of the said assets?
      (ii) What is the Respondent's case as to the value properly to be attributed to his shareholding in the Company? A reasoned valuation by the Company's Accountants or Accountants appointed on the Respondent's behalf in connection with these proceedings is requested, together with copies of any documentation (including but not limited to any valuation by or correspondence with the Share

Valuation by or correspondence with the Share Valuation
Division of the Inland Revenue) which has come into existence during the last three years and which is relevant to the
value of the shares in the Company (for whatever purpose)
during that period.

Reply

(a) Herewith

**(d) (i) Herewith valuation of Valorem & Sons Chartered
Surveyors showing value of £150,000.**

**(ii) Probably on the basis that each share is worth no more
than £4 less than when the Petitioner was repaid her 1%
share. The Respondent's 95% shareholding is therefore
worth approximately £38,000. He is advised that extensive
and costly investigation into the value of the company is
inappropriate (*B* v. *B* 1989 FLR 119) given the known
facts.**

Question

9. Has the Company (or the Respondent personally) received any
offers, approaches or overtures for its acquisition by any person
or by another corporate entity as a going concern? If so, full particulars are requested, together with all documents relating thereto
in the custody, possession or power of the Respondent, including
but not limited to all minutes and memoranda of any board or other
meetings in which the possibility of such flotation has been
disclosed.

Reply

No.

Question

Company (private): directorships generally

10. Give full particulars of all company directorships held by the
Respondent during the last three years.

Reply

None other than in Roberts Engineering Limited.

Question

Credit cards

11. Of what credit, account or charge cards, whether or not in his own name, has the Respondent had the use during the last 3 years? Please produce the statements relating to all such cards to cover the period from 30 September 1994 to the date of answering this Questionnaire (and continuing to the date of trial, unless the Petitioner's Solicitors give notice to the contrary). In the event that any of the items of expenditure appearing on the said statements were reimbursed by the Respondent's company, please mark the statements accordingly.

Reply

Access, Visa and Amex cards. Amex is rarely used. Statements of the other two herewith.

Question

Director's loan account

12. (1) A copy of the Company's private ledger or other documentary record of all movements which have taken place on the Respondent's Director's loan or current account between 30 September 1994 and the date of answering this Questionnaire (and continuing thereafter until the date of trial, unless the Petitioner's Solicitors give notice to the contrary).

(2) Please explain the source and destination of all credit and debit entries respectively which appear in the said ledger or record, insofar as the same are not apparent therefrom.

Reply

The account with the bank suffices to provide a detailed record of the borrowings permitted. Copies of the statements are enclosed showing a balance owing of £40,000.

Question

Holidays, travel abroad generally

13. (1) Copies of the relevant pages of the Respondent's passport to cover the period from June 1994 to the date of answering this Questionnaire.

(2) A schedule of all trips abroad made by the Respondent during this period, stating in respect of each trip:

(a) whether the same was a holiday or in connection with business or both;
(b) by whom the Respondent was accompanied;
(c) the expenditure incurred by the Respondent; and
(d) the source of the funds so expended.

Reply

There have been three trips, one to East Germany for one week of which one day was taken as holiday in Berlin, one to Frankfurt for two days and one for a further trip to Frankfurt for three days. The Respondent was unaccompanied save by a manager from his company and the travel expenditure incurred was paid for by the company save to the extent to which hospitality was provided by the German companies being visited.

Question

Income: company director

14. (1) A schedule of all Director's remuneration, including salary, fees and bonuses received by the Respondent during the last three years.

(2) Does the Respondent have any expectation of an increase in his remuneration during the foreseeable future? If so, please give full particulars.

(3) Copies of the three Forms P11D most recently submitted to the Inland Revenue, together with the accompanying claims under Section 198 of the Income and Corporation Taxes Act 1988.

(4) Please specify all fringe benefits directly or indirectly enjoyable by the Respondent arising out of his employment by the Company, and state precisely to what extent the same are taxed as such by the Inland Revenue.

Reply

(1) See accounts and tax returns
(2) No
(3) Herewith
(4) Car taxed as per Inland Revenue schedule herewith.

Question

Income: tax returns and assessments

15. Copies of the Respondent's Tax Returns and Assessments, with all supporting Schedules referred to therein, in respect of the years of assessment 1992/3, 1993/4 and 1994/5.

Reply

Herewith.

Question

Insurance (life policies)

16. Please produce a schedule of all life insurance policies on the Respondent's life and/or of which he is an actual or potential beneficiary and/or in respect of which he pays or has paid the premiums, giving in the case of each policy the following particulars:
(a) Insurance company;
(b) Policy number;
(c) Type of policy;
(d) Sum assured;
(e) Premiums payable;
(f) Maturity date;
(g) Surrender value (if applicable);
(h) The presently projected sum, inclusive of bonuses, payable upon maturity (if applicable).

Reply

I have one life policy with Marsh Insurance Company number 615293 copy herewith together with statement of its surrender value on the 15 May 1995 (£34,953). The Petitioner is the beneficiary of the policy and it matures in eight years' time.

Question

Investments: stocks and shares, unit trusts etc.

17. (1) If and insofar as this information is not apparent from the Respondent's Tax Returns, a schedule, with dates, of all dealings in stocks, shares, unit trusts and other publicly quoted investments made by the Respondent since 6th April 1994. In the case of any such investment which has either cost or yielded proceeds of sale of or in excess of £6,000, identify the source and destination of the acquisition cost and proceeds of sale respectively.

(2) An up-dated summary prepared by the Respondent's Stockbrokers of his portfolio of investments (to include the base cost in respect of each investment and its yield).

(3) What, according to the Respondent's Accountants, would be the Respondent's liability for capital gains tax if his entire portfolio of investments were disposed of, and how is the same calculated?

Reply

My investments as disclosed, consist of PEPs worth £20,000 for which I enclose the relevant statements. I do not have any investments apart from what I have disclosed. There may be a potential liability to capital gains tax on the sale of the Scottish property but I think it unlikely given the fact that there is unlikely to be any gain.

Question

Land: acquisition or disposal, particulars of

18. In respect of the purchase of Highcroft House please provide completion statement.

Reply

Herewith

Question

Land: mortgaged to bank

19. In respect of the mortgage over 5 Woodside in favour of Gribbins Bank please provide:
(a) A copy of the Mortgage Deed;
(b) A letter from the mortgagee specifying the amount or amounts currently secured by the mortgage, with reference to each and every account (whether presently in credit or debit and whether or not in his own name) which is or may potentially be covered by the security.

Reply

Herewith

Question

Pension arrangements

20 As to the Respondent's self-administered pension scheme please produce:
(a) Documentation showing when it was established;
(b) The value of the funds in which investment has been made;
(c) A statement of the amount which could be allocated to the Petitioner given that she was employed by the Company for three years.

Reply

(a) and (b) herewith. (c) The amount of the Petitioner's potential benefit is very small and the alteration required to the scheme to make her a member of it would I am advised, be disproportionately expensive. Copy letter from my Accountants dated 1 May 1995 herewith.

Question

Tax: principal private residence exemption

21. Please clarify whether the Respondent has elected to treat 5 Woodside as his principal private residence. If so, please produce a copy of the document by which such election was made. What, according to his Accountants, is the position as to the availability of the Extra-Statutory Concession D6?

Reply

The extra-statutory concession will be available until the third anniversary of my absence from the former matrimonial home. I hope that the matter will be resolved before that date.

SERVED by Clements & Co.
on behalf of the Respondent

IN THE PRINCIPAL REGISTRY

No. 3554 of 1994

BETWEEN

ALICE JANE ROBERTS

Petitioner

and

RONALD JAMES ROBERTS

Respondent

REPLIES TO QUESTIONNAIRE OF THE
PETITIONER SERVED ON 15 APRIL 1995
DATED 6 JUNE 1995

Solicitors for the Respondent

IN THE PRINCIPAL REGISTRY   No. 3554 of 1994

BETWEEN

ALICE JANE ROBERTS

Petitioner

and

RONALD JAMES ROBERTS

Respondent

MINUTES OF CONSENT ORDER

UPON the Petitioner and the Respondent agreeing that the provision referred to hereafter is accepted in full and final settlement of all claims the Petitioner and the Respondent may have against each other for capital and property adjustment and other property adjustment including all such claims under the Matrimonial Causes Act 1973 as amended and the Married Women's Property Act 1882.

AND UPON the Petitioner and the Respondent agreeing that their former matrimonial home 5 Woodside, Meadstown, Beamshire registered at HM Land Registry under Title Number BS 753148 shall be transferred to the sole name of the Petitioner subject to the existing mortgage to The Beamshire Building Society

AND UPON the Petitioner and the Respondent agreeing that the with profits endowment policies in their joint names with Lifelong Insurance Company numbered 6921043 and 894762 be transferred into the sole name of the Petitioner.

AND UPON it being further agreed that the parties' home at Highcroft, Measurelyn, Scotland be transferred into the sole name of the Petitioner.

AND UPON the Respondent undertaking that the Petitioner may have the right to inspect at annual intervals beginning with the anniversary of the date of this Order the death in service nomination has made in respect of the policy maintained by the Respondent with Beamshire Insurance Company

AND UPON the Respondent undertaking to the Petitioner on his reaching a pensionable age to give her a lump sum of £25,000 or one quarter of the lump sum payable from his pension scheme with Beamshire Insurance Company whichever shall be larger **PROVIDED THAT** at the date of his death in service or at the date of his retirement the Petitioner shall not have remarried or cohabited with another man for more than three months

AND UPON the Respondent further undertaking that he will not surrender the life policy with Marsh Insurance Company number 615293 of which the Petitioner is the beneficiary

AND UPON the Petitioner and the Respondent agreeing that the contents of the former matrimonial home have been divided in accordance with an agreement between them

AND UPON the parties agreeing that the Petitioner will not seek a variation of the nominal order for periodical payments for herself hereinafter made save in the event of the Respondent becoming unintentionally unemployed

AND UPON the Respondent further undertaking to the court that he will within 14 days from the date of this Order take out with Brokerage Insurance Company a policy of insurance on his life for a term of ten years in the sum of £100,000 (One hundred thousand pounds) for the benefit of the children of the family the Respondent further undertaking to the court to pay all premiums due in respect of the said policy and to do nothing which might prejudice or invalidate the said policy

AND the Petitioner and the Respondent agreeing that all benefits under the said policy whensoever arising shall be paid to the Petitioner or otherwise the children of the family and that neither the Petitioner nor the Respondent shall have any beneficial interest in the policy or its proceeds at any time

AND UPON the Respondent undertaking to the court irrevocably to authorise the said company to release to the Petitioner such information as she may require relating to the policy from time to time but not more frequently than once a year.

BY CONSENT IT IS ORDERED THAT:-

1. The Respondent do transfer to the Petitioner within 14 days of the date hereof the said properties at 5 Woodside, Meadstown subject to the outstanding mortgage to the Beamshire Building Society and Highcroft, Measurelyn, Scotland.
2. As from the date hereof the Respondent do pay or cause to be paid to the Petitioner periodical payments at the rate of 5p per annum during joint lives or until the Petitioner's earlier re-marriage or cohabitation for more than three months or further order whereupon the Petitioner's claims for periodical payments and secured periodical payments do stand dismissed and neither the Petitioner nor the Respondent shall be entitled to make any further application under the Matrimonial Causes Act 1973 Section 23(1)(A) or (B).
3. As from the date hereof the Respondent do pay or cause to be paid periodical payments to the Petitioner for the benefit of each child of the family David born on the 5 September 1978 and John born on the 11 November 1981 until they shall respectively cease full time education or further order at the rate of £35,000 per annum payable monthly in advance.
4. As from the 1 September 1995 the Respondent do pay or cause to be paid to the Petitioner for the benefit of the child of the family John until he shall cease full time secondary education or further order periodical payments of an amount equal to the school fees including the extras in the school bills at the school the said child shall from time to time attend by way of three payments on the 1 September, 1 January and the 1 April of each year.
5. Upon completion of the transfers of the above properties and compliance by the Respondent with his undertakings to the court the Petitioner and the Respondent's claims for lump sum and property adjustment orders do stand dismissed and the Respondent's claims for periodical payments and secured periodical payments do stand dismissed and subject to the terms of clause 2 neither the Petitioner nor the Respondent shall be entitled to make any further application in relation to the marriage under the Matrimonial Causes Act 1973 Section 23(1)(A) or (B).

6. The Respondent do pay the Petitioner's costs of and incidental to this application including the costs of negotiating and implementing this order such costs to be taxed on the standard basis if not agreed.
7. Liberty to apply as to the implementation and timing of the terms of the Order.

Dated the 31 day of August 1995

Signed .Grossfees & Co......... Signed .Clements & Co.........

Solicitors for the Petitioner   Solicitors for the Respondent

References

Booth, Dame Margaret, Maple, G.J., Biggs, A.K., Wall, N. (1991) (eds) *Rayden and Jackson on Divorce and Family Matters* (16th edn), London: Butterworth.

DOE (Department of Environment) (1994) *Department of Environment Code of Guidance in Relation to Homeless Persons*, London: HMSO.

Duckworth, P. (1996) *Matrimonial Property and Finance* (5th edn), London: Longman.

Family Law Bar Association (1994) *At a Glance*, London: Family Law Bar Association.

HMSO (1991) *Family Proceedings Rules*, London: HMSO.

HMSO (1993) *Mediation and the Grounds for Divorce*, London: HMSO.

HMSO (1995) *Improving Child Support*, London: HMSO.

Holloway, D. R. LeB (1993) *Holloway's Probate Handbook* (7th edn), London: Longman.

Howell, Grant (1993) *Family Breakdown and Insolvency*, London: Butterworth.

Law Commission (1988) *Facing the Future*, London: Law Commission.

Law Commission (1990) *The Grounds for Divorce*, London: Law Commission.

Law Society (1991) *Client Care*, London: Law Society.

Law Society (1992) *Enforcement of English Maintenance Orders Abroad*, London: Law Society.

Law Society (1995) *Guide to the Professional Conduct of Solicitors*, London: Law Society.

Leigh, Jane (1992) *The Enforcement of English Maintenance Orders Abroad: A Guide for Solicitors*, London: Family Law Committee of the Law Society.

Mantle, W. (1993) *Child Support: The New System Explained*, London: Longman.

Parker, D, Sax, R. and Rae, P., (1993) *Know How for Family Lawyers* (ed. J. Franklin), London: Longman. [This valuable and detailed work for family practitioners is a useful source of reference on points of law and procedure which the general reader may find of interest.]

Pensions Management Institute (1993) *Pensions and Divorce: Report of the Independent Working Group on Pensions and Divorce Appointed by the Pensions Management Institute in Agreement with the Law Society*, London: Pensions Management Institute.

White, Peter (1995) *Tax Planning on Marriage Breakdown* (5th edn), London: Financial Times.

Organisations and helplines

Association of Consulting
Actuaries
1 Wardrobe Place
London EC4V 5AH
Tel.: 0171 248 3163

Childline
Freepost 1111
London N1 0BR
Freefone 0800 1111

The Children's Legal Centre
20 Compton Terrace
London N1 2NU
Tel.: 0171 359 9392

Dignity
16 Brixham Close
Horston Grange
Nuneaton
CV11 6YT
Tel.: 01203 350312

DSS
RPFA Unit Room 37D
Central Office
Newcastle upon Tyne
NE96 17X

Fair Shares
14 Park Rd
Rugby
Warwickshire CV21 2QH
Tel.: 01788 570585

Family Law Bar Association
Queen Elizabeth Building
Temple
London EC4
Tel.: 0171 583 0497

Family Mediators Association
Tel.: 0181 954 6383

HMSO
High Holborn
London WC1
Tel.: 0171 873 0011

Institute of Actuaries
Staple Inn Hall
High Holborn
London WC1V 7QJ
Tel.: 0171 242 0106

Institute of Family Therapy
43 New Cavendish Street
London W1M 7RG
Tel.: 0171 935 1651

Land Charges Department
Brickhill Court
Burrington Way
Honicknowle
Plymouth
Devon PL5 3LP
Tel.: 01752 635600

Legal Practice
Directorate Information Office
Tel.: 0171 320 5710

Magistrates' Court Division
Lord Chancellor's Department
Trevelyan House
30 Great Peter Street
London SW1 2BY
Tel.: 0171 210 8500

National Family Mediation
(formerly National Association
of Mediation and Conciliation
Services)
Tavistock Place
Tel.: 0171 383 5993

Occupational Pensions Board
PO Box 2EE
Newcastle upon Tyne
NE99 2EE
Tel.: 0191 225 6393

Relate
Herbert Gray College
Little Church Street
Rugby CV21 3AP
Tel.: 01788 573241

Solicitors Family Law
Association
Mrs Mary L'Anson
PO Box 302
Keston
Kent BR2 6EZ
Tel.: 01689 850227

Step Family
72 Willesden Lane
London NW6
Tel.: 0171 372 0844 (enquiries)
0171 372 0846 (helpline)

Tavistock Institute of Marital
Studies
120 Belsize Lane
London NW3 5BA
Tel.: 0171 435 7111

Index

absent parents 4, 99, 101, 105; and housing costs 101; and property and capital settlements 101; and travel to work costs 101–2

acknowledgement of service form 21, 38, 43; example of 182–3

acting for yourself 11, 18, 24

adultery 7, 37, 39, 43, 44; and costs 23

affidavit 21, 23, 44; and financial application 51, 52–4

application for ancillary relief 23, 35, 76, 78, 129, 130; example of 194–217; practice note 150–2; *see also* financial applications

application for dismissal purposes only 40, 130

assets: concealment of 4; and financial application 54–5; removal of abroad 12, 35–6; and setting aside court order 133

attachment of earnings; appeal against 145; order 144–5; and pensions 5; proceedings 144

Attachment of Earnings Act (1971) 144

Attachment of Earnings (Employment Deduction Order) (1991) 145

bankruptcy 61–73; search 61
barristers: use of 19, 55–6, 130

Calderbank offer 24, 50

capital 3, 5, 12, 43, 46, 100, 131, 132, 146; and children 40, 48, 49, 98, 108; and divorce petition 40; and financial claim 52, 56, 57, 59; and judicial separation 29; settlements pre 1993 102

capital gains tax: and the matrimonial home 101, 139, 140–1, 142

case study of divorce 176–221

charging order 148

Charging Orders Act (1979) 146–7

Child Abduction Act (1984) 120

Child Abduction and Custody Act (1985) 120

child benefit 90

Child Support Act (1991) 4–5, 98, 108, 117, 142, 148; and separation agreement 100

Child Support Act (1995) 5, 13, 41, 102, 142

Child Support Agency 4–5, 10, 13, 39, 40, 41, 78, 92–108; and additional expenses 102; appeals against 100, 102, 103,104; and arrears of child maintenance 101, 147–8; and the formula used 105–8; and interim maintenance assessment 104; and people on benefit 104; and protected income 99, 101–2, 107–8; and separation agreement 100